ONE STOP DOC

Immunology

One Stop Doc

Titles in the series include:

Cardiovascular System – Jonathan Aron
Editorial Advisor – Jeremy Ward

Cell and Molecular Biology – Desikan Rangarajan and David Shaw
Editorial Advisor – Barbara Moreland

Endocrine and Reproductive Systems – Caroline Jewels and Alexandra Tillett
Editorial Advisor – Stuart Milligan

Gastrointestinal System – Miruna Canagaratnam
Editorial Advisor – Richard Naftalin

Musculoskeletal System – Wayne Lam, Bassel Zebian and Rishi Aggarwal
Editorial Advisor – Alistair Hunter

Nervous System – Elliott Smock
Editorial Advisor – Clive Coen

Nutrition and Metabolism – Miruna Canagaratnam and David Shaw
Editorial Advisors – Barbara Moreland and Richard Naftalin

Respiratory System – Jo Dartnell and Michelle Ramsay
Editorial Advisor – John Rees

Renal and Urinary System and Electrolyte Balance – Panos Stamoulos and Spyridon Bakalis
Editorial Advisors – Alistair Hunter and Richard Naftalin

Statistics and Epidemiology – Emily Ferenczi and Nina Muirhead
Editorial Advisor – Lucy Carpenter

Coming soon:

Cardiology – Rishi Aggarwal, Emily Ferenczi and Nina Muirhead
Editorial Advisor – Darrell Francis
Volume Editor – Basant Puri

Gastroenterology and Renal Medicine – Reena Popat and Danielle Adebayo
Contributing Author – Thomas Chapman
Editorial Advisor – Stephen Pereira
Volume Editor – Basant Puri

ONE STOP DOC

Immunology

Stephen Boag BMedSci (Hons)
Fifth Year Medical Student, University of Edinburgh, Edinburgh, UK

Amy Sadler BMedSci (Hons)
Third Year Medical Student, University of Edinburgh, Edinburgh, UK

Editorial Advisor: John Stewart BSc PhD
Director of Undergraduate Teaching, School of Biomedical Sciences, University of Edinburgh, Edinburgh, UK

Series Editor: Elliott Smock MB BS BSc (Hons)
Foundation Year 2, University Hospital Lewisham, Lewisham, UK

Hodder Arnold

A MEMBER OF THE HODDER HEADLINE GROUP

First published in Great Britain in 2007 by
Hodder Arnold, an imprint of Hodder Education and a member of the Hodder Headline Group,
338 Euston Road, London NW1 3BH

http://www.hoddereducation.com

© 2007 Edward Arnold (Publishers) Ltd

Whilst the advice and information in this book are believed to be true and
accurate at the date of going to press, neither the author[s] nor the publisher
can accept any legal responsibility or liability for any errors or omissions
that may be made. In particular, (but without limiting the generality of the
preceding disclaimer) every effort has been made to check drug dosages;
however it is still possible that errors have been missed. Furthermore,
dosage schedules are constantly being revised and new side-effects
recognized. For these reasons the reader is strongly urged to consult the
drug companies' printed instructions before administering any of the drugs
recommended in this book.

British Library Cataloguing in Publication Data
A catalogue record for this book is available from the British Library

Library of Congress Cataloging-in-Publication Data
A catalog record for this book is available from the Library of Congress

ISBN 978 0340 92558 4

1 2 3 4 5 6 7 8 9 10

Commissioning Editor: Sara Purdy
Project Editor: Jane Tod
Production Controller: Lindsay Smith
Cover Design: Amina Dudhia
Indexer: Jane Gilbert, Indexing Specialists (UK) Ltd

Typeset in 10/12pt Adobe Garamond/Akzidenz GroteskBE by Servis Filmsetting Ltd, Manchester
Printed and bound in Spain

What do you think about this book? Or any other Hodder Arnold title?
Please visit our website at **www.hoddereducation.com**

CONTENTS

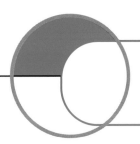

PREFACE

From the Series Editor, Elliott Smock

Are you ready to face your looming exams? If you have done loads of work, then congratulations; we hope this opportunity to practise SAQs, EMQs, MCQs and Problem-based Questions on every part of the core curriculum will help you consolidate what you've learnt and improve your exam technique. If you don't feel ready, don't panic – the One Stop Doc series has all the answers you need to catch up and pass.

There are only a limited number of questions an examiner can throw at a beleaguered student and this text can turn that to your advantage. By getting straight into the heart of the core questions that come up year after year and by giving you the model answers you need, this book will arm you with the knowledge to succeed in your exams. Broken down into logical sections, you can learn all the important facts you need to pass without having to wade through tons of different textbooks when you simply don't have the time. All questions presented here are 'core'; those of the highest importance have been highlighted to allow even shaper focus if time for revision is running out. In addition, to allow you to organize your revision efficiently, questions have been grouped by topic, with answers supported by detailed integrated explanations.

On behalf of all the One Stop Doc authors, I wish you the very best of luck in your exams and hope these books serve you well!

From the Authors, Stephen Boag and Amy Sadler

When we began writing this book, we were aware that immunology has the reputation of being a difficult and 'scary' subject. This did not put us off. Instead, we resolved to write a clear, simple overview of immunology that would be useful to medical students at all stages of their training. We hope we have succeeded in giving you a study tool that makes the complicated parts of immunology easier to understand.

This book is divided into five sections that together provide a complete overview of the immune system, and separately should give you the answers to any specific immunological questions. Immunology is central to the understanding of how the body responds to infection and disease. Therefore, a good grasp of immunology will help you appreciate many concepts central to medicine.

We would like to extend warm thanks to Dr John Stewart who provided tireless advice and encouragement. Thank you also to the team at Hodder Arnold for their help and support.

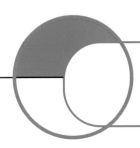

ABBREVIATIONS

ADCC	antibody-dependent cell-mediated cytotoxicity
AICD	activation-induced cell death
AIDS	acquired immunodeficiency syndrome
APC	antigen-presenting cell
ATP	adenosine triphosphate
BALT	bronchial-associated lymphoid tissue
BCR	B cell receptor
C domain/region	constant domain/region
C segment	constant gene segment
CD	cluster of differentiation
CDR	complementarity determining region
CTL	cytotoxic T lymphocyte
CVID	common variable immunodeficiency
DNA	deoxyribonucleic acid
D segment	diversity gene segment
ER	endoplasmic reticulum
Fab	fragment antigen binding
Fc	fragment crystallizable
G-CSF	granulocyte colony-stimulating factor
GM-CSF	granulocyte/monocyte colony-stimulating factor
GVHD	graft-versus-host disease
HEV	high endothelial venule
HIV	human immunodeficiency virus
HLA	human leukocyte antigen
ICAM	intracellular adhesion molecule
IFN	interferon
Ig	immunoglobulin
Ii	invariant chain
IL	interleukin
ITAM	immunoreceptor tyrosine-based activation motifs

J segment	joining gene segment
KIR	killer immunoglobulin-like receptors
LFA-1	leukocyte function-associated antigen
MAC	membrane-attack complex
MALT	mucosal-associated lymphoid tissue
MBL	mannose-binding lectin
M-CSF	monocyte colony-stimulating factor
MHC	major histocompatibility complex
MICA	major histocompatibility complex class I-related chain A
MIIC	MHC class II compartment
mRNA	messenger ribonucleic acid
NADPH	nicotinamide adenine dinucleotide phosphate
NK	natural killer
PAMP	pathogen-associated molecular pattern
PRR	pattern recognition receptor
RAG	recombinase-activating gene
RNA	ribonucleic acid
SCID	severe combined immunodeficiency
TAP	transporter associated with antigen processing
TCR	T cell receptor
T_H1	T-helper type 1
T_H2	T-helper type 2
TLR	Toll-like receptor
TNF	tumour necrosis factor
TSH	thyroid stimulating hormone
V domain/region	variable domain/region
V segment	variable gene segment

INTRODUCTION TO THE IMMUNE SYSTEM

INTRODUCTION TO THE IMMUNE SYSTEM

1. Define the term 'the immune system' and name its two main components

2. With regard to innate immune responses

   a. The innate immune system is more evolutionarily advanced than the acquired immune system
   b. The innate immune system is comprised exclusively of cellular mechanisms
   c. Innate immune mechanisms are dependent on recognition of a specific antigen
   d. The innate immune system recognizes structures shared by different pathogenic microorganisms
   e. Innate immunity can respond rapidly to infection

3. Concerning acquired immune responses

   a. The acquired immune system is dependent on specific recognition of pathogens or pathogen products
   b. The term antigen refers to any molecule that can be recognized by the acquired immune system
   c. Each lymphocyte expresses specific receptors for a wide variety of pathogens on its surface
   d. Before lymphocytes are able to mount an immune response they must recognize an antigen through specific receptors on their surface
   e. Lymphocytes are induced to proliferate following recognition of their specific antigen under appropriate circumstances

4. Categorize the following immune mechanisms or cells as belonging to either the innate (I) or acquired (A) immune system

   a. Phagocytic cells
   b. Antibody
   c. Physical barriers
   d. T cells
   e. Complement
   f. Lysozyme

EXPLANATION: THE IMMUNE SYSTEM – INNATE VS ACQUIRED

The term 'the immune system' refers to the mechanisms that have evolved to protect us from infection (**1**). The immune system has two main components: **innate** and **acquired** immunity (**1**). Both of these utilize **cellular** (direct action of cells) and **humoral** (chemicals secreted into the body fluids) mechanisms.

Innate immunity: The innate immune system consists of a variety of primitive mechanisms to prevent pathogens from gaining access to the body, and early responses to kill the pathogens should they manage to do so. Each response is not specific for a particular pathogen, but can protect the host from a variety of different pathogens by recognizing components found in groups of microorganisms. These defence mechanisms are pre-existing or are generated rapidly. Therefore, they make up the first line of defence against infection.

Mechanisms of innate immunity include physical barriers, such as skin, to stop invading microorganisms, as well as phagocytic cells, such as neutrophils, which ingest and kill pathogens. The humoral component consists of substances, such as lysozyme in tears, and complement in blood and tissue fluids, that are able to kill microorganisms.

Acquired immunity: The acquired immune system is a more evolutionarily advanced system, through which individual pathogens are specifically recognized and immune responses tailored towards them. This branch of the immune system is brought about by leukocytes called **lymphocytes**. Each lymphocyte expresses a receptor on its surface that binds to one specific substance. These substances, which are specifically recognized by the acquired immune system, are known as **antigens**. An antigen can be any type of biological molecule but, for the purposes of protection from infection, many are parts of pathogens or their products. When lymphocytes encounter their specific antigen in the right environment they proliferate and mount an acquired immune response.

The humoral arm of the acquired immune system consists of the production of a substance called **antibody** by a subset of lymphocytes called **B cells**. Antibody molecules bind specifically to antigen and, once bound, facilitate its inactivation or removal. The cellular arm is brought about by another subset of lymphocytes called **T cells**, which help to eliminate pathogens through a variety of mechanisms.

Answers
1. See explanation
2. F F F T T
3. T T F T T
4. a – I, b – A, c – I, d – A, e – I, f – I

5. **Describe each of the following characteristics of the acquired immune responses and outline their importance**

    a. Specificity
    b. Diversity
    c. Memory
    d. Self-regulation
    e. Self/non-self discrimination

6. **Regarding the characteristics of the acquired immune system**

    a. Each lymphocyte expresses a specific receptor that is able to recognize a single epitope
    b. The presence of a vast number of lymphocytes with different specific receptors accounts for the diversity seen in the acquired immune system
    c. The majority of lymphocytes involved in an immune response live on as memory cells
    d. Potentially self-reactive lymphocytes are usually deleted early in their development or inhibited from functioning
    e. Acquired immune responses are downregulated when the stimulus that induced them (i.e. antigen) has been eliminated

EXPLANATION: CHARACTERISTICS OF THE ACQUIRED IMMUNE SYSTEM

The acquired immune system has several important characteristics.

- **Specificity**: acquired immune responses are directed against parts of antigens known as **epitopes** or **antigenic determinants**. This occurs because each lymphocyte can recognize a single epitope through its specific receptor **(5a)**. Under certain circumstances, the lymphocyte responds to the presence of its specific antigen by proliferating and mounting an acquired immune response. This characteristic allows immune responses to be tailored directly towards the pathogen being targeted.
- **Diversity**: each individual possesses a vast number of different lymphocytes, each able to recognize and respond to a specific antigen **(5b)**. Consequently, we are able to mount immune responses to an enormous variety of different pathogens.
- **Memory**: an important characteristic of acquired immune responses is that they improve with repeated exposure to the same pathogen **(5c)**. This occurs because a small number of the lymphocytes involved in the immune response live on as long-lived memory cells. These cells can then mount a more rapid and effective response should re-exposure to the same pathogen occur. This is known as 'immunological memory' and explains why many infectious diseases only affect an individual once in their life (e.g. mumps, chickenpox).
- **Self/non-self discrimination:** it is of vital importance that we only mount immune responses to foreign material and not our own cells **(5e)**. Thus, the immune system must be able to distinguish between self and non-self. The acquired immune system achieves this because any lymphocytes that could potentially recognize self-antigens are eliminated early in their development or are inhibited from functioning. The resulting lack of immune responses to self-antigens is known as **self-tolerance**. This safeguard, however, can sometimes break down, resulting in autoimmune disease.
- **Self-regulation**: there are regulatory mechanisms in place that ensure that the immune response to an antigen is downregulated once the antigen has been eliminated **(5d)**. This prevents energy being expended by continuing immune responses that are no longer required, and allows space for new proliferation of immune cells responding to active infection.

Answers

5. See explanation
6. T T F T T

7. Fill in the blanks in the following paragraph regarding haematopoiesis using the options below (each option can be used once, more than once or not at all)

Options

A. Pleuripotent stem cells

B. Common myeloid progenitor cells

C. Thymus

D. Lymphoid

E. Haematopoiesis

F. Myeloid

G. Bone marrow

The cellular components of blood, including the leukocytes of the immune system, are all derived from a process known as _____, which occurs in the _____. The process begins with _____, which divide and differentiate into the various types of blood cells. The first stage involves differentiation into progenitor cells of two main lineages, known as _____ and _____. These progenitor cells then divide and differentiate further into a wide variety of cell types. Of the lymphocytes, B cells complete their maturation in the _____ and T cells mature in the _____

8. Fill in the blanks in the following diagram showing the process of haematopoiesis

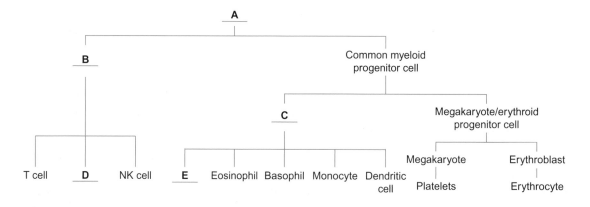

9. Categorize each of the following cell types as being either myeloid (M) or lymphoid (L) in origin

a. Dendritic cells

b. Red blood cells

c. Eosinophils

d. B cells

e. Natural killer cells

NK, natural killer

EXPLANATION: CELLS OF THE IMMUNE SYSTEM – HAEMATOPOIESIS

All of the main cells of the immune system (leukocytes, or white blood cells) originate in the **bone marrow** through a process known as **haematopoiesis**. In this process, **pleuripotent stem cells (8)** divide and differentiate into progressively more specialized and mature cells, which constitute the cellular components of blood. The process is controlled by growth factors, which are produced by the bone marrow stromal cells and the developing blood cells themselves.

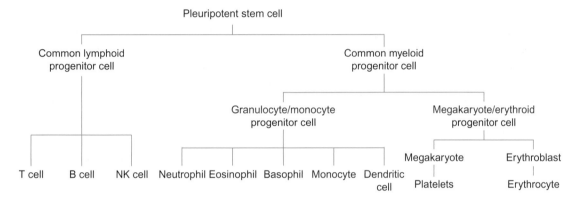

The first step involves the differentiation of pleuripotent stem cells into two cell types: **common myeloid progenitor cells** and **common lymphoid progenitor cells**. At this point, these cells can produce a number of cell types, but are committed to those of either myeloid or lymphoid lineage, respectively.

The common myeloid precursors then differentiate into other precursor cells: **megakaryocyte/erythroid progenitor cells**, which go on to form red blood cells, or erythrocytes, and platelets; and **granulocyte/monocyte progenitor cells**, which go on to form most of the leukocytes of the innate immune system.

The common lymphoid progenitor cells differentiate into the **lymphocytes** that constitute the principal cells of the acquired immune system, and **natural killer (NK) cells**, which represent part of the innate immune system. Of the lymphocytes, **B cells** undergo their entire development in the bone marrow, while lymphoid progenitor cells destined to develop into **T cells** migrate via the bloodstream to the thymus, where they mature.

Answers

7. E, G, A, F, D, G, C
8. A – Pleuripotent stem cell, B – Common lymphoid progenitor cell, C – Granulocyte/monocyte progenitor cell, D – B cell, E – Neutrophil
9. a – M, b – M, c – M, d – L, e – L

10. With regard to phagocytes and antigen-presenting cells

a. Macrophages circulate in the blood, where they are responsible for phagocytosis
b. Antigen presentation to lymphocytes by APCs is an essential step in the initiation of acquired immune responses
c. Neutrophils are specialized cells whose main purpose is antigen presentation
d. The main cells responsible for ingestion and killing of pathogens in infected tissues are macrophages and neutrophils
e. Neutrophils are long-lived cells that reside in the tissues

11. Concerning granulocytes

a. Granulocytes contain cytoplasmic granules rich in toxic substances and inflammatory mediators
b. Eosinophils are responsible for most allergic reactions
c. The main physiological role of eosinophils appears to be in defence against parasites
d. Basophils have a clearly defined role in the protection from most pathogens and are produced in vast numbers in response to infection
e. Mast cells appear to have a role in the acute inflammatory response to infection, through the release of inflammatory mediators, such as histamine

APC, antigen-presenting cell

EXPLANATION: CELLS OF THE IMMUNE SYSTEM – MYELOID CELLS

Dendritic cells: These are specialized cells whose purpose is the presentation of antigen to lymphocytes, an essential step in the initiation of acquired immune responses. They do this by ingesting substances, including pathogens, processing them and presenting fragments on their surface.

Monocytes/macrophages: These are phagocytic cells that are responsible for ingesting and killing pathogens. Monocytes are found in the blood, whereas macrophages develop from monocytes but reside in the tissues. Macrophages are capable of presenting antigen to lymphocytes and, consequently, along with dendritic cells, are known as **antigen-presenting cells** (APCs).

Neutrophils: These are short-lived phagocytic cells that are produced in great numbers in response to infection. They contain cytoplasmic granules rich in toxic substances used to kill pathogens. Owing to the presence of these granules, they are one of a group of cells known as **granulocytes**.

Eosinophils: These are another type of granulocyte with a role in defence against parasites.

Basophils: The precise function of these granulocytes is unknown, although they seem to have a role in inflammation and defence against parasites.

Mast cells: These contain granules rich in inflammatory mediators, including histamine, and are present in most tissues. When activated, they release the contents of these granules into the local environment. They are important cells in acute inflammation and are also responsible for most allergic reactions.

Answers
10. F T F T F
11. T F T F T

12. Regarding B cells and natural killer cells

a. B cells are the only cell type capable of producing antibody
b. Each B cell is only able to produce antibody of a single specificity
c. B cells are activated to produce and release antibody following exposure to their specific antigen
d. NK cells represent part of the acquired immune system
e. NK cells' main role is in defence against intracellular pathogens

13. Considering T cells

a. There are two main classes of T cells, each with different functions
b. Cytotoxic T cells kill self-cells infected with intracellular pathogens
c. Each cytotoxic T cell is able to recognize self-cells infected with a wide variety of pathogens
d. Cytotoxic T cells are responsible for provision of 'help' signals to other immune cells
e. Immune cells provided with 'help' signals from T-helper cells include macrophages and B cells

NK, natural killer

EXPLANATION: CELLS OF THE IMMUNE SYSTEM – LYMPHOID CELLS

Natural killer (NK) cells: These are innate immune cells whose main role is to kill self-cells infected with intracellular pathogens, although they also have a role in killing certain tumour cells

B cells: These are lymphocytes whose main function is antibody production. They are the only cells capable of this and each B cell produces antibody of only one specificity. Production and release of antibody is induced when these cells are activated following exposure to the specific antigen they are able to recognize.

T cells: There are two main classes of these lymphocytes, each with different functions:

- **Cytotoxic T cells** are each able to recognize and kill self-cells that have been infected with a particular intracellular pathogen. They are able to do this as their specific receptor recognizes a fragment of a pathogenic antigen expressed on the surface of host cells. They subsequently respond by killing the host cell and, therefore, the intracellular pathogen within it.
- **T-helper cells** respond to the presence of their specific pathogen by providing signals and factors required to help other immune cells, such as macrophages and B cells, carry out their functions.

Answers
12. T T T F T
13. T T F F T

14. Fill in the blanks in the following statements concerning haematopoiesis using the options listed below (each option can be used once, more than once or not at all)

Options

A. Lymphoid tissues   C. Non-lymphoid
B. Primary   D. Secondary

1. The main tissues involved in the acquired immune system are known as _____
2. _____ lymphoid tissues are the tissues in which lymphocytes develop from lymphoid progenitor cells
3. _____ lymphoid tissues are specialized structures in which acquired immune responses are initiated

15. Categorize the following lymphoid tissues as either primary (P) or secondary (S)

a. Bone marrow   d. Thymus
b. Lymph nodes   e. Spleen
c. MALT

16. With regard to primary lymphoid tissues

a. Developing lymphocytes interact with non-lymphoid cell types in the primary lymphoid tissues
b. Mature T cells are released into the bloodstream from the bone marrow
c. Thymocytes undergo development into mature B cells
d. Thymocytes are surrounded by a network of bone marrow stromal cells
e. The thymus contains bone marrow-derived macrophages and dendritic cells

MALT, mucosal-associated lymphoid tissue

EXPLANATION: TISSUES OF THE IMMUNE SYSTEM

The main tissues involved in acquired immunity are known as lymphoid tissues. These are divided into **primary** (or central) **lymphoid tissues**, where lymphocyte development and maturation occurs, and **secondary** (or peripheral) **lymphoid tissues**, where acquired immune responses are initiated. The primary lymphoid tissues consist of the **bone marrow** and the **thymus**, while the secondary lymphoid tissues consist of the **lymph nodes**, **spleen** and **mucosal-associated lymphoid tissue** (MALT).

Primary lymphoid tissues: These are the sites of lymphocyte development and maturation. In these tissues the developing lymphoid cells are contained within a network of non-lymphoid cells, such as bone marrow stromal cells and thymic epithelial cells. Interactions with these cells are essential in the development of the lymphocytes.

B cells undergo their full development in the bone marrow and are released as mature cells. It is because of their origin in the **bone marrow** that these cells are named **B cells**. The lymphoid progenitor cells that will develop into **T cells**, however, leave the bone marrow early in their development and migrate to the **Thymus**, where they are known as thymocytes.

The thymus is a lobular organ in the upper thorax. Each lobule has a characteristic structure consisting of an **outer cortex** and **inner medulla**, both of which contain large numbers of developing **thymocytes** surrounded by a dense network of **thymic epithelial cells** (see page 63 for a diagram of the thymus structure). Also present are macrophages (throughout the organ) and dendritic cells (confined to the medulla). Within this structure the thymocytes interact with the other cell types and develop into mature T cells.

Answers
14. 1 – A, 2 – B, 3 – D
15. a – P, b – S, c – S, d – P, e – S
16. T F F F T

17. Fill in the blanks in the following statements regarding the role of lymphatics and the lymph nodes in the initiation of immune responses using the options listed below (each option can be used once, more than once or not at all)

Options

A. Effector
B. Lymph
C. Cortex
D. Paracortex
E. Efferent

F. APCs
G. Lymph node
H. Thoracic duct
I. Afferent
J. Lymphatics

1. Extracellular fluid from the tissues drains into a series of vessels known as the _____ This fluid is known as _____ and contains antigen and _____
2. Lymph drains into a _____ from the _____ lymphatics, before passing through the node and back out into the _____ lymphatics, and then into the bloodstream through the _____
3. Lymphocytes constantly circulate between the bloodstream and the lymph nodes, where they form discrete T and B cell zones in the _____ and _____ of the nodes, respectively
4. If a lymphocyte encounters its specific antigen, it is sequestered in the _____, where it proliferates to form _____ cells, which are released and carry out immune responses

18. Concerning the spleen and mucosal-associated lymphoid tissue

a. The lymphoid functions of the spleen are carried out in an area known as the red pulp
b. In addition to lymphoid functions, the spleen is responsible for the destruction of old red blood cells
c. Antigen and APCs enter the spleen via the lymphatics
d. The MALT includes Peyer's patches associated with the gut
e. Antigen is taken up across mucosal surfaces into the MALT by specialized cells known as M cells

APC, antigen-presenting cell; BALT, bronchial-associated lymphoid tissue; MALT, mucosal-associated lymphoid tissue

EXPLANATION: SECONDARY LYMPHOID TISSUES

When pathogens enter the body they are ingested by **antigen-presenting cells** in the tissues. The APCs then migrate to secondary lymphoid tissues. These tissues provide a site where lymphocytes can come into contact with APCs and antigen, allowing initiation of immune responses.

Lymph nodes and lymphatics: The **lymphatics** are vessels into which extracellular fluid drains from the tissues. This fluid (known as **lymph**) contains APCs and antigen. It passes into the **lymph nodes** via the afferent lymphatics. Fluid then leaves the node by the efferent lymphatics, before passing into the blood-stream via the thoracic duct. The APCs, however, stay in the lymph node and present antigen to lympho-cytes. The lymphocytes circulate through the lymph nodes, which they enter from the bloodstream via specialized high endothelial venules. They form discrete T and B cell zones (in the paracortex and cortex of the node, respectively), before draining out via the efferent lymphatics. If lymphocytes are exposed to their specific antigen, they are sequestered in the lymph node, where they proliferate and form effector cells that carry out immune responses.

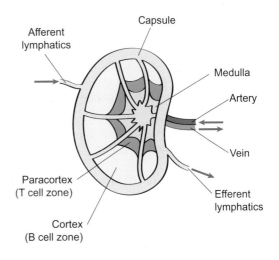

The spleen: The spleen is an abdominal organ which acts as a lymphoid tissue and a site for the destruction of senescent red blood cells. The latter function occurs in the red pulp, whereas the lymphoid functions, which are similar to those of lymph nodes, occur in areas called white pulp. As the spleen has no lymphatic supply, all antigens and APCs enter it via the bloodstream.

Mucosal-associated lymphoid tissue (MALT): This type of secondary lymphoid tissue is associated with mucosal surfaces and includes the tonsils, adenoids, Peyer's patches of the gut, and the bronchial-associated lymphoid tissue (BALT). Antigen is taken up across the mucosal surface by specialized epithelial cells, known as M cells.

Answers
17. 1 – J, B, F; 2 – G, I, E, H; 3 – D, C; 4 – G, A
18. F T F T T

19. Considering the basic characteristics of cytokines

a. Cytokines are usually glycoproteins
b. Cytokines act by binding to specific intracellular receptors and subsequently affecting gene transcription
c. Many cytokines have a large number of different functions
d. Cytokines are uniquely produced by the leukocytes of the immune system
e. Cytokines usually act on the local environment in which they are produced and rarely have effects at distant sites

20. Fill in the blanks in the following statements regarding cytokines using the options below (each option can be used once, more than once or not at all)

Options

A. IL-3	**G.** IL-6
B. G-CSF	**H.** IL-10
C. IL-5	**I.** Monocytes
D. GM-CSF	**J.** TNF
E. Antibody	**K.** Intracellular
F. IL-2	**L.** IFN-γ

1. One cytokine, which acts early in the process of haematopoiesis, is _____; this stimulates development of granuloctye and monocyte precursor cells
2. Other cytokines that act later in this process include _____, which stimulates development of granulocytes specifically, and M-CSF, which similarly stimulates development of _____
3. Another cytokine that acts less selectively to stimulate growth and development of a number of cell types in the bone marrow is _____
4. IL-1, _____ and _____ are examples of cytokines that play an important role in the innate immune response to infection by acting as inflammatory mediators
5. The cytokine profile released by T_H1 cells includes _____, _____ and TNF. These favour development of a cell-mediated response, targeting _____ pathogens
6. The cytokine profile released by T_H2 cells includes IL-4, _____ and _____. These favour development of an _____ response

---

G-CSF, granulocyte colony-stimulating factor; GM-CSF, granulocyte/monocyte colony-stimulating factor; IFN, interferon; IL, interleukin; M-CSF, monocyte colony-stimulating factor; T_H1, T-helper type 1; T_H2, T-helper type 2; TNF, tumour necrosis factor

EXPLANATION: CYTOKINES

Many of the effector mechanisms of the immune system are under the control of secreted molecules known as **cytokines**. These are glycoproteins that are produced and released by many cell types, including fibroblasts, epithelial and endothelial cells, as well as immune cells. They are usually synthesized within these cells in response to a certain stimulus and released into the local environment. They exert their effects by binding to **specific receptors** on the surface of cells and affecting gene transcription. Most individual cytokines are able to act on a number of different cell types and have a variety of effects, often including influencing the production of other cytokines. Many cytokines are produced by a wide variety of different cell types. Furthermore, different cytokines often share similar functions and, consequently, their actions can be described as **redundant**. When cytokines are released, they usually exert their effects locally, affecting both nearby cells and the cell that produced them, but rarely cells at distant sites. Thus they can act in a **paracrine** or **autocrine** fashion (but rarely endocrine).

Certain cytokines have an important role in the production of immune cells by haematopoiesis, and are often known as **colony-stimulating factors** (C_FS). These include **GM-CSF**, which stimulates development of granulocyte and monocyte precursor cells, and **G-CSF** and **M-CSF**, which stimulate development of granulocytes and monocytes, respectively. Others, such as **interleukin-3 (IL-3)**, act as less selective growth factors and encourage proliferation of a variety of cell types in the bone marrow.

The effector mechanisms of innate immunity are often controlled by cytokines. These include **IL-1**, **IL-6** and **tumour necrosis factor (TNF)**, which play a role in inflammation. A variety of cytokines also exert effects on the acquired immune system by controlling activation, growth and differentiation of immune cells. One effect of these cytokines is to tailor the immune response to the type of pathogen being targeted. One cell type that is important in this process is the T-helper (T_H) cell. There are two subsets of this cell type, each of which secretes a different group of cytokines. T_H1 **cells** secrete the cytokines **IL-2**, **interferon-γ (IFN-γ)** and **TNF**, which favour a **cell-mediated** response, appropriate to combat intracellular pathogens. T_H2 **cells**, however, secrete **IL-4**, **IL-5** and **IL-10**, which favour an **antibody** response, better suited to extracellular pathogens.

Answers
19. T F T F T
20. 1 – D; 2 – B, I; 3 – A; 4 – G, J; 5 – F, L, K; 6 – C, H, E

INNATE IMMUNITY

INNATE IMMUNITY

1. Name three types of barrier comprising the initial defence against an invading pathogen

2. Which of the following mechanical barriers act in the gastrointestinal tract?

   a. Tight junctions
   b. Peristalsis
   c. Mucus and cilial action

3. With regard to the basic characteristics of innate defences

   a. Lysozyme is secreted in tears and saliva
   b. Defensins are antimicrobials that breakdown bacterial peptidoglycan
   c. Defensins create a pore in bacterial cell membranes
   d. Cells in the small intestine, respiratory and genitourinary tracts produce defensins
   e. Gastric juices maintain a high pH in the stomach

4. Describe how natural commensal flora acts as an innate defence mechanism

EXPLANATION: INNATE BARRIERS

Host defence against invading pathogens begins at the **epithelial surfaces**, which comprise the skin and the mucosal linings of the respiratory, gastrointestinal and genitourinary tracts. Initially, these epithelial surfaces act as **barriers** to prevent pathogens from entering and colonizing tissues. Barriers can be classed as **mechanical, chemical** or **microbiological**.

- **Mechanical:** Mechanical defences provide **anatomical** or **physical protection** from invading pathogens. For example, continuous loss of dead keratinized cells from the outer epidermis of the skin removes any colonizing microbes. In the gut, **peristalsis** protects against pathogen invasion by propelling the fluid contents swiftly along the tract. Epithelial cells, such as those seen in the gut, are bound together by **tight junctions** that act to seal in the internal environment. In the lung, microorganisms are often expelled in the mucus flow driven by the beating of hair-like cilia found on epithelial cells.
- **Chemical:** Various non-specific antimicrobial chemicals produced by the host play an important role in innate defence. For example, the enzyme **lysozyme** is secreted in both tears and saliva, and acts to degrade bacterial **peptidoglycan**. In the small intestine, paneth cells secrete α-**defensins**, which create a pore in bacterial cell membranes leading to lysis. Related β-**defensins** are secreted by epithelia in the respiratory and genitourinary tracts. In the stomach, gastric juices maintain an acidic pH, which kills microbes.
- **Microbiological**: Non-pathogenic microorganisms found normally within the human body are known as **commensals**. One of the roles performed by commensal microorganisms involves helping to keep potentially harmful pathogens under control (4). For example, commensals may produce antimicrobial substances such as **bacteriocins**. They also **compete** with pathogens for nutrients and epithelial attachment. Commensal organisms are thought to non-specifically **stimulate** the immune system, potentiating a rapid response to an invading pathogen. Their importance is seen when the loss of normal bacterial flora following the use of broad-spectrum antibiotics results in disease. For example, the bacterium *Clostridium difficile* is an opportunistic bacteria normally held in check by natural bacteria flora. However, after antibiotic use, *C. difficile* can overgrow and cause severe pseudomembranous colitis.

Answers

1. Mechanical, chemical and microbiological
2. T T F
3. T F T T F
4. See explanation

5. List three humoral components of the innate immune response

6. Put the following stages involved in the generation of the acute phase response in order

   a. Hepatocytes secrete acute phase proteins
   b. Leukocytes recognize pathogen
   c. Leukocytes release pro-inflammatory mediators, such as interleukin-1 (IL-1), IL-6 and tumour necrosis factor
   d. Pathogen enters body
   e. Pro-inflammatory mediators travel to the liver

7. Name two acute phase proteins and their functions

8. Fill in the blanks in the following statements concerning interferons using the options below (each option can be used once, more than once or not at all)

Options

A. β   **E.** Replication
B. Viral infection   **F.** Stem
C. γ   **G.** α
D. Natural killer

   1. Interferons-α and -β are produced in response to _____
   2. Interferon _____ is produced by virally infected leukocytes
   3. Interferon _____ is produced by virally infected fibroblasts
   4. Interferons inhibit viral _____ and activate _____ cells

IL, interleukin; MBL, mannose-binding lectin; NK, natural killer; TNF, tumour necrosis factor

EXPLANATION: HUMORAL COMPONENTS

The innate immune response has a humoral arm that consists of circulating soluble substances.

Acute phase proteins: During acute illness, activated leukocytes release **pro-inflammatory mediators**, such as tumour necrosis factor, interleukin-1 (IL-1) and IL-6, in response to recognition of invading microorganisms. These mediators travel to the **liver** and stimulate the synthesis and secretion of proteins, termed acute phase proteins, by hepatocytes. Well-characterized acute phase proteins include C-reactive protein and mannose-binding lectin (MBL). **C-reactive protein** facilitates the attachment of microbial surface antigens to phagocytic cells, thus enhancing phagocytosis. Such substances are known as **opsonins**. C-reactive protein is also known to activate the complement system, which in turn promotes inflammation and pathogen destruction. MBL also activates complement via a different pathway.

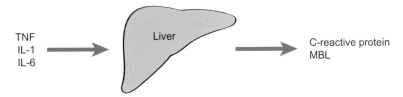

Interferons α and β (INF-α and -β): These mediators are released by **virally infected** cells in response to the presence of double-stranded viral RNA. INF-α and -β are characteristically produced by leukocytes and fibroblasts, respectively. Upon binding to a surface receptor on an uninfected cell, the interferons induce a state of **viral resistance**. For example, they act to inhibit viral replication and can activate natural killer (NK) cells.

Complement: The complement system consists of **circulating plasma proteins** present in blood and tissue fluids. They are activated to perform various mechanisms associated with innate immune defences.

Answers

5. Acute phase proteins, interferons and complement
6. d, b, c, e, a
7. C-reactive protein, mannose-binding lectin; see explanation for functions
8. 1 – B, 2 – G, 3 – A, 4 – E, D

9. Name three different pathways of complement activation

10. Match the pathways below to the following statements

Options

    A. Classical pathway
    B. Mannose-binding lectin pathway
    C. Alternative pathway

    1. This is activated by recognition of microbial carbohydrates
    2. This is activated by antigen-antibody complexes
    3. This is activated by spontaneous hydrolysis of C3

11. Concerning complement pathways

    a. Mannose-binding lectin recognizes bacterial mannose residues
    b. The classical pathway involves the spontaneous hydrolysis of C3
    c. All three pathways result in the formation of C3 convertase
    d. The alternative pathway occurs on pathogen surfaces
    e. The classical pathway can be activated by direct recognition of pathogen surfaces

MBL, mannose-binding lectin

EXPLANATION: COMPLEMENT PATHWAYS

Complement proteins are present in an inactive form but can be activated to provide many effector functions of inflammation and humoral immunity. There are known to be three different pathways through which the complement system can be activated, all ending in a common amplifying enzyme cascade.

The classical pathway: This is activated principally by the binding of the complement component **C1** to an **antigen–antibody complex**. This indicates that an adaptive immune response is required to initiate this innate defence mechanism. However, there is also evidence that the pathway can be directly activated by the **surface components** of certain pathogens, such as retroviruses and *Mycoplasma*.

The mannose-binding lectin (MBL) pathway: In this case, initiation is via the binding of MBL to a specific **spatial** arrangement of microbial carbohydrates that include **mannose** and **fucose**.

The alternative pathway: This differs from the previous two pathways in that activation involves the **spontaneous hydrolysis** of the complement component C3. Usually, the cascade is prevented by the action of specific **regulatory proteins** found on host cell surfaces. However, no such proteins are found on pathogens, and the alternative pathway can proceed on the **pathogen surface**.

All three pathways involve a series of reactions that result in the formation of an enzyme called a **C3 convertase**. The production of this enzyme represents the convergence of the pathways and the generation of the main effector functions of complement.

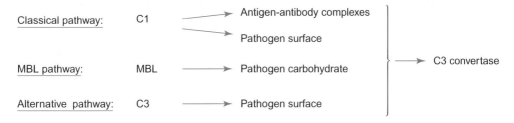

Classical pathway: C1 → Antigen-antibody complexes
→ Pathogen surface

MBL pathway: MBL → Pathogen carbohydrate

Alternative pathway: C3 → Pathogen surface

→ C3 convertase

Answers

9. Classical, mannose-binding lectin and alternative
10. 1 – B, 2 – A, 3 – C
11. T F T T T

12. Considering complement

a. C5 convertase is formed from C5a and C5b
b. C5 convertase is formed from C3b and C3 convertase
c. C3a and C3b are formed by C5 convertase
d. The membrane-attack complex consists of C5b, C6, C7, C8 and C9

13. Name four innate defence functions carried out by complement proteins

14. Which complement proteins can be termed anaphylatoxins?

15. Match the complement proteins below to the following statements

Options

A. C3a
B. C5a
C. C3b
D. C5b

1. It triggers inflammation
2. It is part of the membrane-attack complex
3. It is a chemoattractant
4. It can act as an opsonin

MAC, membrane-attack complex

EXPLANATION: COMPLEMENT FUNCTION

The three complement pathways converge with the production of the enzyme **C3 convertase**. This cleaves the component C3 into two further components named **C3a** and **C3b**. C3a is released but C3b is bound to the target pathogen membrane. C3b binds the original C3 convertase to form a **C5 convertase**, a complex that cleaves the complement component C5 into C5a and C5b. C5b, on the pathogen surface, subsequently binds the complement components C6, C7, C8 and C9 to form the **membrane-attack complex (MAC)**, which spans the pathogen plasma membrane forming a **pore**. Importantly, a series of regulatory proteins ensures that complement does not damage normal host cells.

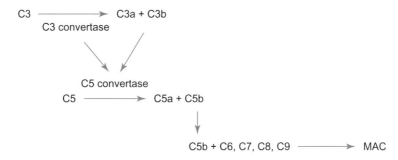

The various complement proteins carry out four main innate defence functions:

1. **Triggering inflammation** – C5a, and to a lesser extent C3a and C4a, promote **inflammation**. They act to stimulate smooth muscle **contraction** and increase vascular **permeability**. In addition, C5a and C3a bind to receptors on mast cells and basophils, and induce the release of pro-inflammatory mediators, such as **histamine**. When present at a high level, these complement fragments are involved in a generalized circulatory collapse termed anaphylactic shock and are, therefore, termed **anaphylatoxins.**
2. **Attraction of immune cells** – C5a also functions as a **chemoattractant** for neutrophils and monocytes by increasing their migration towards the site of infection.
3. **Opsonization** – C3b and to a lesser extent, C4b can act as **opsonins** by potentiating the attachment of microbes to complement receptors on phagocytic cells.
4. **Pathogen lysis** – the MAC is a doughnut-shaped structure with a hydrophobic exterior that allows association with the pathogen membrane. Its internal hydrophilic channel acts as a pore in the lipid bilayer and results in loss of membrane integrity and eventual **destruction** of the pathogen.

Answers

12. F T F T
13. Inflammation, chemoattraction, opsonization and pathogen lysis
14. C3a and C5a
15. 1 – A, B; 2 – D; 3 – B; 4 – C

16. How does the innate immune system distinguish between self and non-self?

17. Answer the following questions about innate recognition of microorganisms

    a. What are PAMPs?
    b. Name three characteristics of PAMPs
    c. List three examples of PAMPs
    d. What name is given to host receptors that recognize PAMPs?
    e. What are TLRs?

18. Complete the following table concerning Toll-like receptors

TLR	Location	Target
TLR4	A	B
C	D	Unmethylated CpG DNA

19. Name another pattern-recognition receptor (not of the Toll-like receptor family) and describe its role in innate defences

DNA, deoxyribonucleic acid; MBL, mannose-binding lectin; PAMP, pathogen-associated molecular pattern; PRR, pattern-recognition receptor; RNA, ribonucleic acid; TLR, Toll-like receptor

EXPLANATION: PATTERN RECOGNITION RECEPTORS

The innate immune system demonstrates **broad specificity** characterized by the ability to distinguish self from non-self. This involves receptors that activate innate defences following recognition of molecules present on invading pathogens, but not present within the host **(16)**.

Microorganisms typically contain molecular motifs known as **pathogen-associated molecular patterns** or PAMPs **(17a)**. PAMPs are invariant within a pathogen class, essential for pathogen survival and not seen as part of the normal host **(17b)**. Well-characterized PAMPs include **lipopolysaccharide** present in Gram-negative bacterial cells walls, unmethylated repeats of CpG present in bacterial DNA and **double-stranded RNA** seen in viral infection **(17c)**.

Innate receptors that recognize PAMPs are termed **pattern-recognition receptors** or PRRs **(17d)**. PRR ligation can initiate various effector functions including **phagocytosis** and secretion of mediators, such as **cytokines**.

The best-characterized family of PRRs is the **Toll-like receptor** family (TLR) **(17e)**. For all TLRs, ligation triggers a series of protein cascades that leads to the activation of transcription factors including **NFκB**, which in turn activate genes encoding various proteins involved in immune defence. In mammals, TLR4 is found on the surface of macrophages and dendritic cells, and recognizes bacterial lipopolysaccharide. Another TLR, TLR9, is found intracellularly in the same cells and recognizes unmethylated CpG DNA.

An example of a secreted PRR is **mannose-binding lectin** (MBL), previously mentioned as an activator of complement **(19)**.

Answers

16. See explanation
17. See explanation
18. A – Surface of macrophages and dendritic cells, B – Lipopolysaccharide, C – TLR9, D – Within macrophages and dendritic cells
19. See explanation

20. Name two types of phagocytic cell

21. Place the following steps involved in phagocytosis in the correct order

a. Pseudopod formation
b. Pathogen destruction
c. Actin polymerization and depolymerization
d. PAMP recognition
e. Phagosome formation
f. Phagolysosome formation

22. Fill in the blanks in the following statements concerning the mechanisms of pathogen destruction using the options below (each option can be used once, more than once or not at all)

Options

A. Burst
B. Cytoplasmic membranes
C. Peptidoglycan
D. Dependent
E. Lactoferrin
F. Independent

1. Lysozyme breaks down _____. It is oxygen-_____
2. NADPH oxidase formation requires a respiratory _____
3. Cationic proteins disrupt _____
4. _____ prevents microbial use of iron

23. How do salmonella and mycobacteria avoid phagocyte destruction?

NADPH, nicotinamide adenine dinucleotide phosphate; PAMP, pathogen-associated molecular pattern; PRR, pattern recognition receptor

EXPLANATION: PHAGOCYTES

Innate immunity also includes a cellular component. The **phagocytes** comprise one of the most important innate cell groups. These include **monocytes**, which migrate from the circulation to the body tissues to become mature **macrophages**, and **neutrophils**. Phagocytes can internalize and kill many pathogens.

The process of phagocytosis begins with cellular expression of various surface PRRs that are specific for PAMPs. These include scavenger receptors and a receptor that recognizes bacterial lipopolysaccharide, called CD14. Enhanced recognition and attachment of the phagocyte to a microbe is achieved in the presence of an **opsonin**, e.g. the complement fragment C3b or antibody. Following attachment, actin polymerization and depolymerization within the phagocyte leads to the formation of **pseudopods** of cytoplasm and membrane that engulf the microbe to form a **phagosome**. The phagosome then fuses with one or more intracellular granules called lysosomes to form a **phagolysosome**. Lysosomes contain antimicrobial enzymes and proteins that can destroy the pathogen. Pathogen destruction in the phagolysosome can be further classified as oxygen-dependent and oxygen-independent.

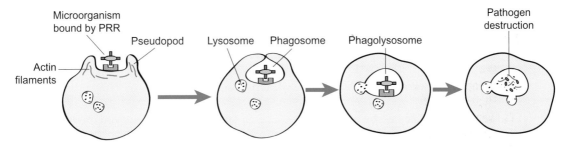

- **Oxygen-dependent**: Phagocytosis stimulates a respiratory burst accompanied by a transient increase in oxygen consumption. This generates an NADPH oxidase, which converts oxygen into the damaging **superoxide anion** (O_2^-). Further reactions produce a range of **antimicrobial chemicals** including hydrogen peroxide (H_2O_2) and hydroxyl radicals ($OH\cdot$).
- **Oxygen-independent**: Many lysosomes contain **cationic proteins** that disrupt cytoplasmic membranes, **lysozyme**, which breaks down peptidoglycan, **lactoferrin**, which deprives bacteria of iron, and various other antimicrobial enzymes.

Some bacteria are relatively resistant to phagocytic destruction. For example, some species of salmonella prevent fusion of the phagosome with the lysosome **(23)**. Pathogenic mycobacteria have been shown to inhibit the acidification of the phagosome required for lysosomal enzyme action **(23)**.

Answers

20. Neutrophils, monocytes (become macrophages)
21. d, c, a, e, f, b
22. 1 – C, F; 2 – A; 3 – B; 4 – E
23. See explanation

24. Concerning natural killer cells

   a. They are of lymphoid origin
   b. They contain intracellular granules
   c. They are vital in containing viral infection
   d. They are triggered by inhibitory receptors only
   e. They bind membrane components of host cells

25. Name two methods of natural killer cell recognition and activation

26. Fill in the blanks in the following statements considering natural killer cells using the options below (each option can be used once, more than once or not at all)

Options

   A. Cytotoxicity
   B. IL-12
   C. IL-1
   D. Antibody secretion

   E. TNF
   F. IFN-γ
   G. Interferons
   H. Opsonization

   1. Natural killer cells can be activated by _____ and macrophage-derived mediators including _____ and _____
   2. Activated natural killer cells demonstrate _____ and secrete _____

27. Regarding natural killer cell killing

   a. It requires both perforin and granzymes
   b. Perforin binds a mannose-6-phosphate receptor
   c. Perforin binds phosphorylcholine
   d. Perforin creates a pore in the target cell membrane
   e. Granzymes activate proteolytic enzymes called caspases

IFN, interferon; IL, interleukin; KIR, killer immunoglobulin-like receptor; MAC, membrane-attack complex; MHC, major histocompatability complex; MICA, major histocompatability complex class I-related chain A; NK, natural killer; TNF, tumour necrosis factor

EXPLANATION: NATURAL KILLER CELLS

Natural killer (NK) cells are **large lymphoid cells** with prominent **cytoplasmic granules** and considerable **cytotoxic** activity. They are known to be vital in containing viral infection by acting to remove virally infected host cells. NK cell killing is dependent upon the interaction of both inhibitory and activating NK receptors that bind components of the host cell surfaces. NK cells are activated by recognition of 'altered self' and 'missing self'.

- **Altered self** refers to the change in cell surface components that results from viral infection. For example, the cell may upregulate expression of **stress molecules**, such as MICA (major histocompatibility complex class I-related chain A), which in turn bind activating NK cell receptors and result in infected cell death.
- **Missing self** refers to the absence of normal cell surface components that results from viral infection. For example, normal expression of a major histocompatibility complex (MHC) class I molecule acts via a set of inhibitory NK-cell surface receptors called **KIRs (killer immunoglobulin-like receptors)** to prevent NK-mediated killing. Viral infection may lead to downregulation or prevention of MHC class I expression on the infected cell surface. This will lead to loss of KIR inhibition and NK-mediated killing of the infected cell.

Initially, NK cells can be activated in response to interferons and macrophage-derived factors including **IL-12** and **TNF**. Besides cytotoxic action, this activation stimulates NK cell secretion of large levels of **IFN-γ**. IFN-γ has **antiviral properties** and in turn is vital in the **activation of macrophages**.

NK cell cytotoxicity is dependent on the combined action of **perforin** and **granzymes**, both found within NK cell granules. Perforin binds **phosphorylcholine** on the target cell membrane and polymerizes to form a pore similar to that seen in the complement MAC. Granzymes were originally believed to enter the target cell via the pore formed by perforin. However, it now appears that granzymes bind first to a cell surface receptor for mannose-6-phosphate. Upon entry, they activate a **proteolytic cascade** involving enzymes called **caspases**. This also triggers cell death.

Answers
24. T T T F T
25. Missing self and altered self
26. 1 – G, E, B; 2 – A, F
27. T F T T T

28. List the five signs of inflammation

29. Considering inflammation

    a. Prostaglandins are released during mast cell degranulation
    b. Inflammatory mediators cause local vasodilation
    c. Redness and heat are caused by increased blood supply to inflamed tissues
    d. Inflammatory mediators cause decreased vascular permeability
    e. Fluid leaking into inflamed tissues causes swelling and contributes to the pain experienced

30. List three functions of the inflammatory exudate

31. Regarding the outcomes of inflammation

    a. Phagocytic cells are attracted into inflamed tissues by the release of chemotactic agents
    b. IL-8 acts as a chemotactic factor in inflammation
    c. Neutrophils and monocytes are responsible for ingestion and removal of the causative agent in inflammation
    d. Neutrophils play an important role in stimulating tissue repair at the conclusion of inflammation
    e. Inflammation usually results in a permanent impairment of tissue function

IL, interleukin

EXPLANATION: INFLAMMATION

Inflammation is the response of the body to any form of tissue injury, which can be due to infection, exposure to toxic substances or physical trauma. The characteristic signs of inflammation are **redness, heat, swelling, pain** and **loss of function**. The process is brought about by the release of a variety of inflammatory mediators. The three main effects of these are **vasodilation, increased vascular permeability** and **cellular infiltration** into the tissue.

The key event in the initiation of inflammation is **mast cell degranulation**, which results in the release of several inflammatory mediators, including vasoactive **amines**, such as **histamine** and **5-hydroxytryptamine**. Various other cell types also produce a variety of inflammatory mediators, such as prostaglandins and leukotrienes. These mediators cause local vasodilation, increasing the blood supply to the tissue, causing the characteristic redness and heat. This is beneficial as it increases the supply of the cells and substances required to combat the causative insult.

Inflammatory mediators also cause increased vascular permeability, allowing fluid and proteins to leak into the tissue, resulting in swelling and pain (owing to increased tissue tension). Mediators, such as prostaglandins and kinins, also have a direct action on nerves and cause pain. The functions of this **exudate** include the supply of important substances, such as clotting factors and fibrin, which is deposited and acts as a barrier to the spread of any invading microorganisms **(30)**. Other useful substances in the exudate include **immunoglobulins** and **complement proteins**. Furthermore, the inflammatory exudate also serves to dilute any toxic substances present in the tissue, as well as carrying antigen to the lymph nodes by draining into the lymphatics **(30)**.

The other main function of the inflammatory mediators are to act as chemotactic agents, attracting inflammatory cells into the tissue. Important chemotactic mediators include: **leukotrienes, complement component C5a** and several **cytokines** (e.g. IL-8). The cells attracted include neutrophils and monocytes, which are able to ingest and remove the causative agent. Once this has been successfully done, certain cells, including monocytes, then stimulate repair of the damaged tissue. In most circumstances this resolution returns the tissue to its previous state of function.

Answers

28. Redness, heat, swelling, pain and loss of function
29. F T T F T
30. See explanation
31. T T T F F

ACQUIRED IMMUNITY

ACQUIRED IMMUNITY

1. Label the following diagram of an antibody molecule

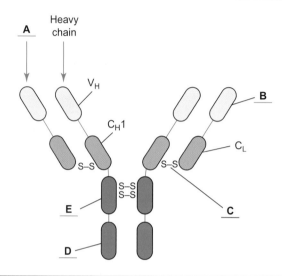

2. With regard to antibody structure

a. The two heavy chains in an antibody molecule are bound together by covalent disulphide bonds
b. Weak non-covalent interactions bind the heavy chains to the light chains
c. Each heavy chain consists of one variable domain and one constant domain
d. The variable domains of the two light chains are aligned to form the antigen-binding site
e. All heavy chains consist of a variable domain and at least three constant domains

3. Name two other molecules of the Ig gene superfamily that are involved in the processes of antigen presentation and recognition

4. Considering the component parts of an antibody molecule

a. The protease papain divides the antibody molecule into one Fc portion and two Fab portions by bisecting the heavy chains
b. The Fc component of an antibody molecule is comprised entirely of parts of the two heavy chains
c. The Fc component confers specificity upon an antibody
d. The Fab component contains the variable domains of both heavy and light chains
e. The Fc component has no effect on the function of the antibody molecule

---

Fab, fragment antigen binding; Fc, fragment crystallizable; Ig, immunoglobulin

EXPLANATION: ANTIBODY STRUCTURE

Antibodies, or immunoglobulins (Ig), are **glycoproteins** that constitute the main humoral component of the acquired immune system and carry out their functions by binding to a specific antigen. Despite the enormous variety of antibody specificities, all antibody molecules share the same basic structure. They are composed of four glycoprotein chains: two identical **heavy chains** and two identical **light chains (1)**. The heavy chains are covalently bound together by **disulphide bonds (1)**, and one light chain is covalently bound to each heavy chain, giving the Y-shaped molecule shown below.

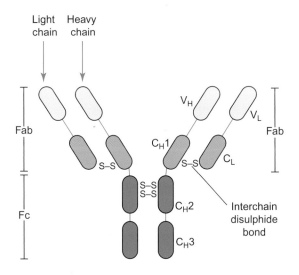

Each of the chains is composed of a number of similar structures, known as **domains**, of approximately 110 amino acids in length. Each domain is arranged in a characteristic globular conformation known as an **Ig fold**. This is formed by the polypeptide folding into two adjacent β-pleated sheets held together by intrachain disulphide bonds. Such structures are seen in a variety of other molecules, collectively referred to as the **immunoglobulin gene superfamily**. These include other molecules involved in antigen presentation and recognition (e.g. major histocompatibility complex molecules and T cell receptor) as well other cell surface molecules (e.g. CD4, CD8)

Each light chain in an antibody molecule consists of two domains, **one variable domain** (V_L) and **one constant domain** (C_L). The heavy chains are each composed of **one variable domain** (V_H) and **three or four constant domains** (C_H1, C_H2, C_H3 and sometimes C_H4) **(1)**.

Proteases that cleave antibodies can provide information about the functions of the different parts of the molecule. The protease papain splits antibody molecules into two **Fab** fragments (each made up of a light chain and the V_H and C_H1 heavy-chain domains) and an **Fc** fragment (made up of the remaining domains of the two heavy chains). The Fab fragments are responsible for **antigen binding**, while the Fc fragment determines other features of the molecule's function.

Answers

1. A – Light chain, B – V_L, C – Disulphide bonds, D – C_H3, E – C_H2
2. T F F F T
3. Major histocompatibility complex molecules and T cell receptor
4. T T F T F

5. Regarding the antigen-binding site (paratope)

a. Each monomeric antibody molecule possesses one site for antigen binding

b. The site for antigen binding is formed by the variable domains of both the heavy and light chains

c. The variable domains of the heavy and light chains vary between antibody molecules of different specificity

d. There are six areas in each variable domain that show particularly high variability and determine an antibody's specificity

e. The antigen-binding site is formed by three CDRs from a V_H domain and three from a V_L domain

6. Concerning the epitope and paratope

a. The antigen-binding site on an antibody is also known as the epitope

b. The area on an antigen to which an antibody binds is known as the paratope

c. When an antibody binds its antigen, the epitope and paratope are held together tightly by covalent bonds

d. In order for an epitope and paratope to bind, they must fit closely together

e. The interactions that bind the paratope to the epitope are weak and are only effective over very short distances

7. True or false? Each of the following types of interactions contributes to binding of the epitope to the paratope

a. van der Waals forces

b. Disulphide bonds

c. Hydrophobic interactions

d. Hydrogen bonds

e. Electrostatic interactions

CDR, complementarity determining region; V domain, variable domain

EXPLANATION: ANTIGEN BINDING BY ANTIBODY

Each monomeric antibody molecule is able to bind to its specific antigen via two **antigen-binding sites**. These sites are formed by the V_H and V_L domains, in which there is variability in the amino-acid sequence between antibodies of different specificities.

Within each of the two V domains (V_H and V_L) there are **three separate amino-acid sequences** that show most variability. The antibody molecule is folded in such a way as to bring these six hypervariable segments into alignment to form the antigen-binding site, or **paratope**. These areas determine the specificity of the antibody and are consequently known as **complementarity determining regions** (CDRs).

Given that an antigen can be any kind of biological molecule, it is likely that most will be far larger than the binding site on an antibody. Consequently, antibodies tend only to bind to a small part of the antigen. The specific area on the antigen that is bound by an antibody is known as the **epitope** or **antigenic determinant**. Non-covalent binding of the epitope to the paratope is achieved through a variety of mechanisms including: electrostatic interactions, hydrogen bonds, van der Waals forces and hydrophobic interactions. These individual interactions are weak and, therefore, only act over very short distances. Consequently, the epitope and paratope must fit tightly together to allow the forces to act strongly enough to facilitate strong binding.

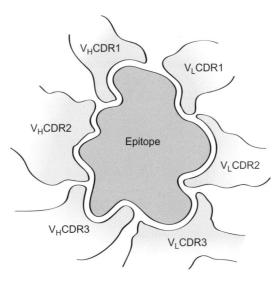

8. Use the options below to fill in the blanks in the following paragraph concerning antibody isotypes (each option can be used once, more than once or not at all)

Options

A. Alpha
B. Two
C. Heavy
D. IgG
E. IgE
F. Five
G. Delta

H. Seven
I. IgM
J. IgD
K. Light
L. Nine
M. IgA

The biological functions of an antibody molecule, with the exception of antigen binding, are determined by the _____ chain. There are _____ main types of this chain, which results in the same number of antibody classes. Of these classes, _____ and_____, are further divided into subclasses, owing to slight variations in the _____ chains

9. Considering different types of antibody molecule

a. Antibody molecules can be produced in membrane-bound or secreted forms
b. Secreted antibody molecules have a hydrophobic terminating sequence
c. There are two different types of light chain, known as κ or λ chains
d. An antibody molecule can contain one κ light chain and one λ light chain
e. There is no known difference in the function of κ and λ light chains

---

C domain/region, constant domain/region; Ig, immunoglobulin

EXPLANATION: ANTIBODY ISOTYPES I

The biological functions of antibodies are largely determined by the heavy chain. In humans there are five main heavy-chain types – α, δ, ε, γ and μ – and these result in five **classes**, or **isotypes**, of antibody – IgA, IgD, IgE, IgG and IgM, respectively. Of these classes, IgA and IgG are further divided into **subclasses**, each with subtly different heavy-chain C regions.

Antibody molecules can be produced in **secreted** or **membrane-bound** forms, depending on the terminating sequence of the heavy-chain C regions. The membrane-bound form terminates with hydrophobic residues that anchor it in the plasma membrane, while the secreted form lacks these residues.

In addition to the different heavy-chain classes, there are two different types of light chain, known as **kappa** (κ) and **lambda** (λ) **chains**. Each antibody molecule contains light chains of one of these types, but not both. These chains differ in their C domains, but there are no known differences in the function of antibodies with κ or λ light chains.

Answers

8. C, F, M, D, C
9. T F T F T

10. Fill in the class of antibody to which each of the following statements refer

a. _____ is the most abundant class of antibody in the extramucosal tissues of the body

b. _____ is further subdivided into four subclasses, each with slightly different heavy chains and effector functions

c. _____ and _____ are found as membrane-bound receptors for antigen on the surface of naive B cells

d. _____ is found bound to the surface of mast cells and is responsible for mediating allergic reactions

e. _____ is further subdivided into two subclasses, each with slightly different heavy chains and effector functions

f. _____ is primarily found in the blood as a pentamer of five antibody molecules

g. _____ is the most abundant class of antibody in the mucosal tissues of the body

h. _____ is the only class of antibody capable of crossing the human placenta into the fetal circulation

i. _____ can be found as a dimer of two antibody molecules linked by a polypeptide known as a J-chain

BCR, B cell receptor; C domain/region, constant domain/region; Fc, fragment crystallizable; Ig, immunoglobulin

EXPLANATION: ANTIBODY ISOTYPES II

IgA is the most abundant class in the secretions of the body's **mucosal surfaces**. It is further divided into two subclasses, IgA1 and IgA2, with subtly different heavy-chain C regions. The secreted form is found as a **dimer** of two antibody molecules linked by a polypeptide J-chain.

IgD is almost exclusively found as a membrane-bound molecule on the surface of naive **B cells** in the periphery, where, along with IgM, it acts as the receptor for antigen recognition.

IgE is a class of antibody found on the plasma membrane of **mast cells**, **basophils** and, at times, **eosinophils**, where it is bound by a receptor for its Fc portion. When cross-linked by antigen, it induces degranulation, causing release of **inflammatory mediators**. This process has a role in initiating acute inflammation and allergic reactions. The heavy chains of IgE antibodies consist of five domains (one variable and four constant domains). Levels of IgE are elevated in asthma.

IgG is the most abundant class of antibody in the **blood** and **extramucosal tissues** of the body. In addition to its role in the mature immune system, it is the only class of antibody to cross the human placenta into the fetal circulation. It is divided into four subclasses: IgG1, IgG2, IgG3 and IgG4.

IgM is the first type of antibody produced in an immune response. It is found primarily in the **blood** as a **pentamer** of five identical antibody molecules, each of which has heavy chains composed of five domains. It is also found as single antibody molecules on the surface of naive **B cells**, where it acts as an antigen receptor (B cell receptor; BCR).

Answers

10. a – IgG, b – IgG, c – IgM and IgD, d – IgE, e – IgA, f – IgM, g – IgA, h – IgG, i – IgA

11. Put the following statements regarding the generation of heavy-chain diversity in the correct order

a. The DNA encoding the heavy chain is transcribed to produce a primary mRNA transcript
b. The recombinase enzyme complex joins a random D segment to a J segment
c. The DNA for a random V segment is joined to the DJ segment
d. The final mRNA encoding the heavy chain is translated to produce the polypeptide chain
e. The mRNA encoding the variable domain (VDJ segments) is joined to that encoding the constant domains (C segments) by mRNA splicing

12. With regard to antibody gene rearrangement

a. There are two separate areas of the genome that encode different types of light chains
b. The variable domain of a light chain is made up of the products of three recombined gene segments: a V, a D and a J segment
c. Within a light-chain locus, any V segment can potentially be joined to any J segment
d. The recombination of germline DNA to produce the DNA encoding antibodies occurs in developing B cells in the bone marrow
e. Considerable heavy-chain diversity is ensured by the random joining of V, D and J gene segments, as there are a huge number of potential combinations

---

C segment, constant gene segment; DNA, deoxyribonucleic acid; D segment, diversity gene segment; Ig, immunoglobulin; J segment, joining gene segment; mRNA, messenger ribonucleic acid; RNA, ribonucleic acid; V segment, variable gene segment

EXPLANATION: GENERATION OF ANTIBODY DIVERSITY I

The enormous diversity of antibody molecules is achieved primarily by rearrangement of the germline DNA. This DNA is found in three loci of the genome, one encoding the heavy chain (on chromosome 14), and two encoding the different types of light chains, κ and λ (chromosomes 2 and 22, respectively).

The light-chain variable domain (V_L) is the product of two gene segments: a **V** (**variable**) **segment** and a **J** (**joining**) **segment**. The germline DNA contains a number of potential gene segments for each of these (40 V and 5 J segments in the case of the κ chain locus). Early in B cell development, one of each of these gene segments are randomly selected and brought together through the action of a **recombinase** enzyme complex to produce the DNA encoding a V_L domain. This process is known as **somatic recombination**. The recombined DNA encoding the entire light chain is then transcribed to produce a primary transcript mRNA. The VJ region of this transcript is then joined to the **C** **segment** encoding the constant domains, in a process known as **splicing**. This resultant VJC mRNA strand is translated to produce the light chain. The random joining of the V and J segments ensures considerable light-chain diversity, as there are a large number of potential combinations.

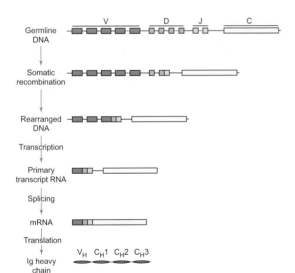

The process is similar for the heavy-chain locus. However, as well as V and J segments, there are also **D** (**diversity**) **segments** in the germline DNA. The recombinase joins a D segment to a J segment, and the resultant DJ segment to a V segment. The heavy-chain locus contains 51 V, 27 D and 6 J segments, ensuring enormous diversity in the heavy chains produced. The rearranged DNA is then transcribed to produce a primary transcript mRNA. The VDJ section of this transcript is then joined to the **C segment** that encodes the constant domains. This mRNA is then translated into the heavy-chain product. This method of generating antibody diversity is known as **combinatorial diversity**.

Answers

11. b, c, a, e, d
12. T F T T T

13. Concerning mechanisms for the generation of antibody diversity

a. Any two B cells that produce the same heavy chain must produce antibodies with the same specificity

b. The potential to combine any possible heavy chain with any possible light chain contributes to antibody diversity

c. The recombinase enzyme complex is extremely accurate in aligning the appropriate sequences when joining gene segments together

d. Slight inaccuracies in gene segment joining by the recombinase complex have no effect on antibody specificity

e. There is a high rate of somatic mutations in the DNA encoding the antibody CDRs in mature, activated B cells

14. Match the following options to the appropriate method of ensuring antibody diversity:

Options

A. Combinatorial diversity
B. Junctional diversity
C. Affinity maturation

1. Two B cells produce identical light chains but different heavy chains. The two cells produce antibodies specific for different antigens

2. A somatic mutation in the DNA encoding one of the antibody CDRs occurs during division of an activated B cell. The change results in production of a slightly different antibody, with a higher affinity for its antigen

3. Two developing B cells join the same V and J segments when recombining their DNA to produce an antibody light chain. However, in one of the B cells the recombinase complex includes an extra nucleotide in the join. Consequently, the two cells produce different light chains

CDR, complementarity determining region; DNA, deoxyribonucleic acid; D segment, diversity gene segment; J segment, joining gene segment; V segment, variable gene segment

EXPLANATION: GENERATION OF ANTIBODY DIVERSITY II

Another type of **combinatorial diversity** that contributes to the vast array of antibody specificities in an individual stems from the fact that both the heavy and light chains contribute to the specificity, but their genes are rearranged independently. Consequently, any heavy chain can potentially be **combined** with any light chain. This means that more than one B cell can, for instance, make the same heavy chain but combine it with a different light chain, producing an antibody with a different specificity.

Another method in place to maximize antibody diversity is through imprecision in the joining of the V, D and J segments, and is known as **junctional diversity**. The recombinase enzyme complex, responsible for breaking, realigning and joining the DNA, is inaccurate and can include or exclude nucleotides on either side of the intended join. This can result in changes in the amino-acid sequence of the resultant variable domain and, consequently, a different antibody specificity.

Finally, still more antibody diversity is achieved in mature B cells. During an immune response there is a tendency for **somatic mutations** to occur in the DNA encoding the hypervariable regions of antibody molecules in activated, dividing B cells. The resultant changes in the amino acid sequences of the CDRs alter the antibody's affinity for antigen, effectively producing a slightly different antibody molecule. Some of these B cells will produce antibody with increased affinity for the antigen that the immune response is directed against. These cells are **positively selected**, resulting in an overall increase in the affinity of antibody for antigen as an immune response progresses. This process is known as **affinity maturation**, and is discussed further on page 55.

Answers

13. F T F F T
14. 1 – A, 2 – C, 3 – B

15. Considering antibody production and gene rearrangement

a. B cells are each able to produce only one specificity of antibody

b. The germline DNA for each B cell contains two heavy-chain alleles and four light-chain alleles

c. A mature B cell can produce up to two different heavy chains and four different light chains

d. All antibody gene rearrangements result in the production of a viable gene product.

e. Developing B cells that do not successfully rearrange their genes to produce a viable antibody molecule die before reaching full maturity

16. Put the following statements in this example of allelic exclusion in the correct order

a. When rearrangement of the first heavy-chain allele is unsuccessful, rearrangement begins on the other allele

b. Rearrangement of the light-chain κ alleles occurs in turn but fails to result in production of a viable light chain

c. Rearrangement of the second heavy-chain allele is successful and heavy-chain gene rearrangement stops

d. An immature B cell begins rearranging its germline DNA by recombining the gene segments on one of its heavy-chain alleles

e. The B cell begins to produce its complete antibody molecule as the heavy and light chains are combined

f. Rearrangement begins on the first light-chain λ allele. This results in production of a viable light chain

g. Rearrangement of light-chain genes is stopped and does not proceed to the second λ allele

DNA, deoxyribonucleic acid

EXPLANATION: ALLELIC EXCLUSION

Each B cell is able to produce antibody of one specificity. However, there are three areas of the genome that encode parts of an antibody molecule, and we have a diploid genome with two alleles of each gene. Each B cell, therefore, possesses the DNA to carry out somatic recombination enough times to produce **two** different heavy chains and **four** different light chains (two κ and two λ). This is of potential benefit because not all gene rearrangements are successful and result in formation of a viable gene product. The presence of more than one allele for each type of chain, therefore, increases the likelihood of a developing B cell successfully being able to produce a viable heavy chain and light chain. In reality, however, each B cell is only ever able to produce one heavy chain and one light chain, ensuring its single specificity. This is ensured by the ordered rearrangement of the genes, in a process known as **allelic exclusion**.

The rearrangement of a B cell's germline DNA begins with one of its heavy-chain alleles. If this is successful and results in a viable product, heavy-chain gene rearrangement stops and the other allele is not used. If it is unsuccessful, gene rearrangement starts on the other allele. If this too is unsuccessful, then the B cell will not go on to produce a viable antibody molecule and is induced to die by **apoptosis**. However, if a heavy chain is successfully produced, gene rearrangement starts on the light-chain loci, initially on one κ allele. If this is successful, then gene rearrangement stops and the B cell produces its antibody. However, if it is unsuccessful, gene rearrangement begins on the other κ allele, followed in turn by each of the λ alleles, if required. Consequently, only one heavy chain and one light chain are produced, ensuring a single antibody specificity.

Answers

15. T T F F T
16. d, a, c, b, f, g, e

17. **Label each phase of antibody production in the graph below and describe what is happening**

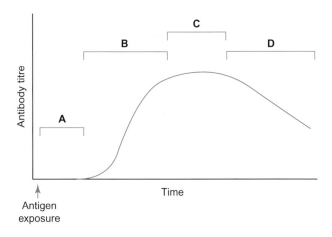

18. **Put the following statements regarding the generation of antibody responses in the correct order**

    a. The B cell undergoes clonal expansion and differentiates to produce plasma cells capable of producing large quantities of antibody
    b. When a B cell encounters its specific antigen in a lymph node, the B cell's surface receptors bind the antigen and the cell is sequestered in the lymph node
    c. A T-helper cell, specific for the same antigen, binds antigen:MHC complexes on the surface of the B cell, and provides it with help
    d. The antigen bound to the B cell's receptors is internalized, processed and presented on the cell surface by MHC class II molecules
    e. Naive B cells expressing surface IgM and IgD circulate between the bloodstream and secondary lymphoid tissues

19. **Regarding antibody production**

    a. Naive B cells are incapable of producing antibody for secretion
    b. Ligation of B cell receptors by specific antigen is usually sufficient to activate the cell
    c. All T cells express CD40L, regardless of their activation status
    d. The interactions between T and B cells that result in the generation of antibody responses occur in the secondary lymphoid tissues

Ig, immunoglobulin; IL, interleukin; MHC, major histocompatibility complex; TCR, T cell receptor

EXPLANATION: ANTIBODY PRODUCTION I

Antibody production follows a consistent pattern, with four distinct phases. Initially, there is a **lag phase** during which the levels of antibody (or titre) in the serum are undetectable while the processes required for antibody production get under way. This is followed by a **log phase** in which there is a rapid rise in the antibody titre. There is then a **plateau phase**, during which the titre remains fairly constant. Finally, there is a **decline phase** during which the antibody response is downregulated and antigen–antibody complexes are removed from the serum.

Initial antibody production: Production of antibody for secretion requires a B cell to be activated through binding of its surface immunoglobulin (Ig) by antigen. For most antigens there is also the requirement for another signal, supplied by an activated T-helper cell responding to the same antigen. This is known as **linked recognition**.

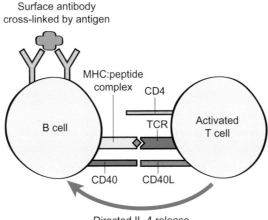

When a B cell encounters its antigen, some of its ligated surface Ig is internalized, allowing the antigen to be processed and presented on the cell surface by MHC class II molecules (see page 75). If these are then bound by an activated T-helper cell, the B cell is provided with the additional help signals required for activation. One such signal is the ligation of CD40 molecules on the B cell surface by **CD40L**, which is expressed by activated T-helper cells. (For simplicity, in the diagram, only one of each molecule is shown. In reality, there are many of each.)

The T cell also releases **cytokines**, including interleukin-4 (IL-4), which cause the B cell to proliferate and form **plasma cells**. These plasma cells produce secreted antibody, initially of the IgM class. The initial interaction between B and T cells occurs at the edge of the T-cell zone in secondary lymphoid tissues, where the proliferating cells form an area of clonal expansion known as a **primary focus**.

Answers

17. A – Lag phase, B – Log phase, C – Plateau phase, D – Decline phase
18. e, b, d, c, a
19. T F F T

20. Fill in the blanks in the following paragraph regarding antibody production in germinal centres using the options below (each option can be used once, more than once or not at all)

Options

A. Primary focus

B. Primary lymphoid follicle

C. Affinity maturation

D. Class switching

E. Follicular dendritic cells

F. Germinal centre

Some of the B cells formed in the initial primary focus in a secondary lymphoid tissue subsequently migrate into a _____. Here they rapidly divide and set up an area of proliferation known as a _____. This area contains rapidly dividing B cells, as well as _____. Within this area, the B cells undergo various processes including: _____, which results in an increased antibody affinity for antigen, and _____, which results in production of different antibody classes

21. Concerning class switching

a. Different antibody classes have different heavy-chain constant domains that are encoded separately within the heavy-chain locus

b. Antibody class switching occurs in B cells within the primary focus

c. Antibody class switching involves rearrangement of the heavy-chain DNA

d. The class of antibody produced after class switching is influenced by the cytokines to which the B cell is exposed

e. Once class switching has occurred, the B cell is unable to switch back to production of IgM

22. Explain the process of affinity maturation, by which the affinity of antibody for antigen increases throughout an immune response

CDR, complementarity determining region; DNA, deoxyribonucleic acid; Ig, immunoglobulin

EXPLANATION: ANTIBODY PRODUCTION II

Following the initial phase of B cell proliferation and formation of plasma cells, some of the B cells in the primary focus migrate into a **primary lymphoid follicle**, where they set up another zone of proliferation known as a **germinal centre**. Here they interact with specialized cells known as **follicular dendritic cells**, and undergo the processes of affinity maturation and class switching.

Class switching: The various antibody classes have different heavy-chain constant domains, each encoded by separate genes within the heavy-chain locus. B cells in the germinal centres are able to rearrange their DNA in order to produce heavy chains of these types. This involves positioning the desired C gene next to the genes encoding the variable domain and removal of the intervening DNA. As the intervening genes are removed, class switching cannot be reversed but can continue until the final C gene (that encoding IgA2 constant domains) is used. The C gene selected during class switching is determined by the cytokines to which the cell is exposed.

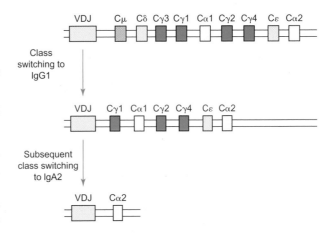

Affinity maturation (22): Throughout an immune response, the average affinity of antibodies for antigen increases over time. This is because the dividing B cells in the germinal centre undergo a high rate of point mutations in the DNA encoding the antibody CDRs. This can result in progeny whose antibody has altered affinity for antigen. If antibody affinity is increased, the cells become better able to bind and internalize antigen and present it to T cells. As a result, they are better able to compete with other B cells for the survival signals provided by T cell help. Consequently, B cells with desirable mutations are positively selected and go on to proliferate further. This occurs with each generation of B cells, resulting in a progressive increase in affinity of antibody for antigen.

Answers

20. B, F, E, C, D
21. T F T T T
22. See explanation

23. With regard to antibody effector functions

a. The process by which some antibodies are able to prevent pathogens from adhering to and infecting host cells is known as opsonization

b. Neutralization is dependent on antibodies binding to parts of an antigen important for its function

c. Antibodies are often able to prevent damage to host tissues by bacterial toxins through the process of neutralization

d. The effector function of neutralization is conferred upon an antibody by its Fc portion

e. Toxin neutralization by antibody can be an important immune defence mechanism

24. Considering complement activation by antibody

a. The main way in which antibodies activate complement is through initiating the alternative complement cascade

b. The C1q portion of the C1 complex is activated by binding the Fc portion of IgD or IgE

c. The activation of C1q is dependent on cross-linking by binding two Fc portions

d. The activation of complement results in the recruitment of phagocytes

e. One important consequence of complement activation is lysis of the pathogen

25. In relation to opsonization and antibody-dependent cell-mediated cytotoxicity

a. An opsonin is a substance that when bound to a pathogen increases the ability of phagocytes to ingest and kill it

b. Fc receptors on the surface of phagocytes only signal and induce phagocytosis when cross-linked by antibody bound to antigen

c. The complement component C3b can act as an opsonin

d. ADCC involves the ingestion of infected host cells by phagocytes

e. NK cells are able to kill large pathogens or infected host cells through ADCC

ADCC, antibody-dependent cell-mediated cytotoxicity; Fc, fragment crystallizable; Ig, immunoglobulin; NK, natural killer

EXPLANATION: ANTIBODY EFFECTOR FUNCTIONS

Once an antibody has bound to its antigen, it can perform a number of functions that assist in the removal or inactivation of the antigen.

Neutralization: This involves the antibody binding to biologically important parts of the antigen and preventing it carrying out its function. If antibody binds to an important residue on a bacterial toxin, for instance, the toxin can be **neutralized**, preventing damage to the host. Furthermore, many viruses and bacteria are dependent on molecules on their surface to allow them to adhere to host cells. Antibodies that bind these molecules will prevent the pathogen from being able to infect host cells.

Complement activation: The complement component **C1q** is able to bind to the Fc portion of IgG or IgM when they are bound to antigen. When C1q is cross-linked by two Fc portions, it becomes activated, setting off the **classical complement cascade**. This has several effects, including inducing an inflammatory response, bringing phagocytes to the area and causing lysis of microorganisms through the formation of the **membrane-attack complex**.

Opsonization: Antibodies can act as **opsonins**, meaning that they can greatly increase the ability of **phagocytes** to ingest and kill pathogens. A variety of phagocytes express surface receptors for antibody Fc portions. Importantly, these receptors only signal to the cell when they are cross-linked, therefore limiting this to occasions when they bind multiple antibodies bound to the surface of a pathogen, rather than free antibody. The resultant signal induces the phagocyte to ingest and kill the microorganism. Furthermore, some components of the classical **complement** cascade (such as C3b), which can be initiated by antibody, also act as opsonins.

Antibody-dependent cell-mediated cytotoxicity (ADCC): This involves the use of antibody to induce the killing of infected host cells or pathogens too large for phagocytosis. This occurs when Fc receptors on the surface of some immune cells, such as natural killer (NK) cells or macrophages, are cross-linked by antibody bound to antigen. The immune cell is induced to release **toxic substances** into the space between the two cells, killing the target cell.

Answers
23. F T T F T
24. F F T T T
25. T T T F T

26. Concerning monoclonal antibodies

    a. When individuals are immunized with a single antigen, they respond by producing antibody of one specificity

    b. It is impossible to obtain a pure sample of a single specificity of antibody from the serum of an individual

    c. A monoclonal antibody is a pure sample of identical antibody molecules with a single specificity

    d. A sample of monoclonal antibody consists exclusively of the antibody produced from the progeny of an individual hybridoma cell

    e. Monoclonal antibodies are always produced by hybridoma cells formed by fusing human B cells with human myeloma cells

27. Put the following statements about the technique for producing monoclonal antibodies in the correct order

    a. Individual hybridoma cells are cultured in wells and the supernatants tested for the presence of the desired antibody

    b. The cells from wells containing the desired antibody are cultured indefinitely, producing a constant pure supply of the desired monoclonal antibody

    c. The B cells are fused with myeloma cells to give them the ability to divide indefinitely, producing hybridoma cells

    d. The mixture of B cells, myeloma cells and hybridoma cells are cultured in HAT medium, in which, after a few cycles of cell division, only the hybridoma cells survive

    e. A suspension of cells containing antibody-producing B cells is produced from the spleen of the mouse

    f. A mouse is immunized with the antigen against which a pure sample of specific antibodies is desired

28. List four uses of monoclonal antibodies in either research or clinical medicine

EXPLANATION: MONOCLONAL ANTIBODIES

When an animal is immunized with an antigen, it produces a variety of antibodies specific for all possible epitopes within the antigen. It is, therefore, impossible to obtain a pure sample of a specific antibody from the serum. However, it can be useful for immunologists to produce a large number of identical antibody molecules with a known specificity. These are known as **monoclonal antibodies** and a technique has been developed for producing these.

The process involves taking **B cells** from the spleen of a mouse immunized with the desired antigen. These cells cannot be cultured indefinitely, as normal B cells are programmed to die after a certain number of divisions. Consequently, the normal B cells have to be fused with **myeloma cells**, which do not produce any antibody themselves but, as they are cancer cells, have lost the control mechanisms that prevent them from proliferating indefinitely. The resultant fused cells are known as **hybridomas** and produce antibody while being able to divide indefinitely. The cells are cultured in a medium (known as HAT medium) in which the unfused myeloma cells are unable to survive. Given the tendency for the normal B cells to die within a small number of cell divisions, after a few cycles, only the hybridoma cells remain. These cells are then cultured individually in wells, so that each well contains the progeny of a single cell. The supernatant from each well is tested for the presence of the desired antibody. The cells from a well yielding a positive result are cultured indefinitely and the antibody produced collected. This antibody is known to be monoclonal (as it is produced by the progeny of a single hybridoma cell) and has the desired specificity.

Monoclonal antibodies have a wide range of uses both clinically and in research **(28)**. They can be used for the **identification** and **classification** of cell types based on the surface molecules they express, as well as in blood typing. They are also useful in analysing the **function** of biological molecules, for instance, cell surface receptors, by blocking or stimulating them. In addition, they can be helpful in the **diagnosis** of disease through the detection of antigens or antibodies. They are also being used increasingly, and with some success, in attempts to treat or prevent disease.

Answers

26. F T T T F
27. f, e, c, d, a, b
28. See explanation

29. Answer the following questions about B cell development

    a. Which cell type present in the bone marrow is required for B cell development?
    b. Describe two ways in which they provide help

30. Place the following statements about B cell development in order

    a. Heavy-chain immunoglobulin rearrangement
    b. Surrogate light chain combined with heavy chain
    c. IgM expression
    d. Light-chain immunoglobulin rearrangement
    e. B cell progenitor produced in bone marrow

31. Put the following B cell types in order of maturation (least mature to most mature)

    a. Immature B cell
    b. Pro-B cell
    c. Small pre-B cell
    d. Lymphoid progenitor cell
    e. Large pre-B cell

Ig, immunoglobulin

EXPLANATION: B CELL DEVELOPMENT

B cell development occurs when lymphoid progenitor cells in the bone marrow receive signals from non-lymphoid **stromal cells** also present in the bone marrow. The stromal cells secrete factors that promote B cell differentiation, such as the chemokine **CXCL12**, and additionally provide **adhesive contact** for the developing cells **(29b)**.

The earliest B cells are called **pro-B cells**. In these cells, rearrangement of the immunoglobulin heavy-chain locus occurs as already discussed. Successful expression of viable μ chains means these cells can then be classed as **pre-B cells**. In pre-B cells, the μ chains are seen in combination with a surrogate light chain and together form a membrane structure called a **pre-B cell receptor**. The surrogate light chains structurally resemble actual light chains but are identical on every pre-B cell. At this point, cells are known as **large pre-B cells**. Successful expression of the pre-B cell receptor halts recombination at the heavy-chain loci and the cell undergoes several rounds of proliferation. The resulting cells are known as **small pre-B cells**. In the small pre-B cell, the immunoglobulin light chain undergoes rearrangement. Successful assembly of a light chain then allows surface expression of a complete **IgM** molecule, the antigen receptor for the B cell. The cell is now known as an **immature B cell**.

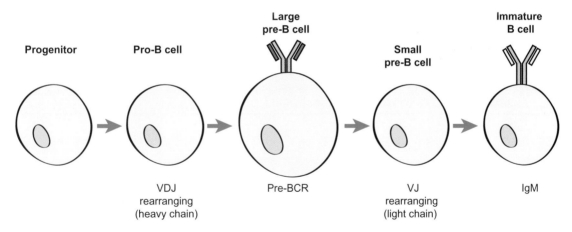

Once an immature B cell expresses surface IgM, its fate is determined by its ability to bind to self-molecules present in the bone marrow. A similar process is seen in T cells in the thymus. As with T cells, the resulting B cell repertoire, ready to exit to the periphery, should thus be **tolerant** to self-antigens. The mechanisms are explained elsewhere (see page 95).

Answers

29. a – Stromal cells, b – See explanation
30. e, a, b, d, c
31. d, b, e, c, a

32. Name four different cell types found in the thymus

33. Explain the importance of thymic epithelial cells in T cell development

34. Fill in the blanks in the following statements concerning T cell development using the options below (each option can be used once, more than once or not at all)

Options

A. Medulla

B. Puberty

C. Macrophages

D. Adulthood

E. Thymocytes

F. Cortex

1. Immature T cells in the thymus are known as _____
2. The greatest rate of thymic T cell production is seen before _____
3. Immature thymocytes are seen in the _____ of the thymus
4. Thymocytes that are nearly mature are seen in the _____ of the thymus

35. What percentage of thymocytes survive passage through the thymus? Why do a proportion of thymocytes die in the thymus?

CD, cluster of differentiation; TCR, T cell receptor

EXPLANATION: T CELL DEVELOPMENT I

T cells, in common with B cells, arise from common lymphoid **precursor** cells found in the **bone marrow**. Precursor cells destined to become T cells selectively migrate to the **thymus**, where they are known as **thymocytes**.

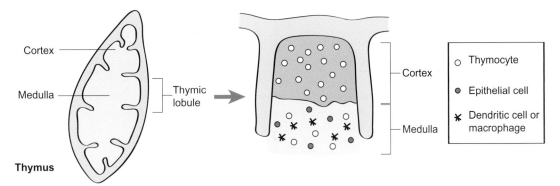

The thymocytes are found within a network of epithelia called the thymic **stroma**. Other cells present in the thymic medulla include dendritic cells and macrophages. The importance of thymic epithelial cells is illustrated in mice with a mutation in a transcription factor required for thymic epithelial differentiation **(33)**. These mice have no thymus and a severe deficiency in T cell numbers. The greatest rate of T cell production by a normal thymus is seen before **puberty** and, in humans, the role of the thymus in adulthood is much debated. Recently migrated immature thymocytes are found mainly in the outer **cortex** of the thymus. Within the inner thymic **medulla**, T cells at a more mature stage of development are seen. Interestingly, most of the immature T cells (about 98 per cent) die within the thymus indicating a very **high selection pressure**.

Developing thymocytes undergo a series of changes characterized by the expression of different surface molecules including the T cell receptor (TCR) and co-receptors, named CD4 and CD8. Cell-surface molecules such as CD4 and CD8 are designated CD (or cluster of differentiation) based on recognition by a group of monoclonal antibodies.

Answers

32. Thymocytes, epithelial cells, macrophages and dendritic cells
33. See explanation
34. 1 – E, 2 – B, 3 – F, 4 – A
35. Approximately 2 per cent, high selection pressure

36. Answer the following questions using options from the list below (each option can be used once, more than once or not at all)

Options

A. V

B. RAG

C. J

D. β

E. MHC class III genes

F. D

G. α

1. Name the genes vital for the genetic rearrangement of the TCR
2. Which gene segments are involved in rearrangement of the TCR α-chain?
3. Which gene segments are involved in rearrangement of the TCR β-chain?
4. Rearrangement of this chain occurs at the double-negative stage of T cell development
5. Rearrangement of this chain occurs at the double-positive stage of T cell development

37. Regarding γδ T cells

a. They comprise the majority of the T cell population
b. These cells might not express surface CD4 or CD8
c. They all recognize the antigen associated with MHC molecules
d. They are found in high levels within epithelia
e. Their precise function is not known

CD, cluster of differentiation; MHC, major histocompatibility complex; RAG, recombinase-activating gene; TCR, T cell receptor

EXPLANATION: T CELL DEVELOPMENT II

Recently migrated thymocytes are classed as 'double-negative', as they express neither of the surface co-receptors known as CD4 or CD8. At this point, genetic rearrangement of the T cell receptor (TCR) chains analogous to the rearrangement of the immunoglobulin heavy-chain locus occurs. The process is dependent on **recombinase-activating gene** (RAG) products. As seen in antibodies, TCR genes are assembled from V, D and J region segments by **genetic recombination**. This process gives rise to the huge diversity of receptor specificity seen in the T cell population.

Most T cells have receptors composed of chains designated α and β. The β-chain is assembled from V, D and J segments at the **double-negative stage** of development when thymocytes express neither CD4 nor CD8. Production of this β-chain allows association with a surrogate α-chain to form a **pre-T cell receptor**, analogous to the pre-B cell receptor discussed previously. Successful expression of the pre-T cell receptor switches off RAG expression, stimulates proliferation and moves the cell into the **double-positive stage** of maturation where both CD4 and CD8 are expressed. At this stage, RAG genes are switched back on and act to rearrange the α-chain locus, which involves only V and J segments. Successful production of an α-chain allows thymocyte expression of a complete surface TCR.

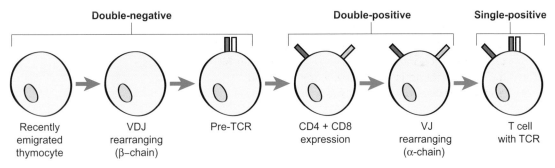

A minority of T cells bear receptors with chains designated γ and δ. These T cells differ from T cells expressing α and β-chain receptors in that their receptor is encoded by different gene segments, and CD4 or CD8 might not be expressed on their surface. Additionally, they recognize a variety of different antigens, and do not normally require antigen presentation by MHC class I or class II molecules (see page 69). The $\gamma\delta$ T cells are found in high levels within **epithelia** but their precise function remains unknown.

Answers

36. 1 – B; 2 – A, C; 3 – A, C, F; 4 – D; 5 – G
37. F T F T T

38. Using the information on the opposite page and pages 63 and 65 arrange the following events in T cell development in the order in which they occur

    a. Positive selection
    b. Double-negative cells
    c. Migration of common lymphoid precursors from the bone marrow to the thymus
    d. Double-positive cells
    e. Negative selection

39. Regarding T cell development

    a. Positive and negative selection both rely on MHC expression
    b. Cells that fail to bind self-peptide:MHC complexes survive
    c. Cells that bind self-peptide:MHC complexes with a very high affinity survive
    d. Cells that reach the periphery have a low affinity for self-peptide:MHC complexes
    e. Many cells die during positive and negative selection

MHC, major histocompatibility complex; TCR, T cell receptor

EXPLANATION: T CELL DEVELOPMENT III

Maturation in the thymus is completed when double-positive cells expressing surface T cell receptors undergo two processes known as **positive and negative selection**. Both processes rely on recognition of **major histo-compatibility complex (MHC) molecules** expressed on the surface of thymic epithelial cells and other antigen-presenting cells present in the thymus. These MHC molecules bind **self-peptides** and present them to developing T cells.

Positive selection of the T cell repertoire involves successful recognition of self-peptide:self-MHC complexes by developing T cells. Thymocytes that have no affinity for the complexes die by **apoptosis**. Positive selection thus determines survival of cells expressing T cell receptors (TCRs) that can bind specific MHC molecules. These cells become **single-positive**: if an MHC class I molecule is recognized, surface CD8 is retained, and if an MHC class II molecule is recognized, CD4 is retained.

Surviving cells then undergo negative selection. This involves the elimination of potentially harmful self-reactive cells that recognize self-peptide:MHC with too high an affinity. Negative selection contributes to **immune tolerance,** whereby the immune system does not respond to self-antigens. The result is a population of mature, albeit naive, CD4 or CD8 single-positive thymocytes, which have a low affinity for self-MHC but which will **not be self-reactive** in the periphery. Most cells do not survive both positive and negative selection.

Answers
38. c, b, d, a, e
39. T F F T T

40. Describe why the MHC is vital for effective immune responses

41. Fill in the blanks in the following sentences using the options below (each option can be used once, more than once or not at all)

Options

A. HLA-DR
B. HLA
C. HLA-A
D. Hetero
E. HLA-C
F. II
G. HLA-B

H. Haplotype
I. Six
J. 17
K. I
L. Homo
M. HLA-DP
N. HLA-DQ

1. The human MHC is located on chromosome _____.
2. Human MHC genes involved in antigen presentation are called _____ genes.
3. MHC class I genes are called _____, _____ and _____.
4. HLA-DR, HLA-DP and HLA-DQ are MHC class _____ genes.
5. Most individuals are _____zygous for MHC.
6. MHC genes are expressed co-dominantly meaning most individuals express at least _____ molecules of each class.
7. The MHC _____ is the combination of MHC genes on one chromosome in an individual

42. Complete the following table

MHC molecule class	Distribution	Recognized by T cell subset
I	A	B
II	C	D

43. List two molecules encoded by MHC class III genes

HLA, human leukocyte antigen; MHC, major histocompatibility complex; TNF, tumour necrosis factor

EXPLANATION: MAJOR HISTOCOMPATIBILITY COMPLEX

The major histocompatibility complex (MHC) comprises a linked set of highly **polymorphic genes** that encode a set of membrane **glycoproteins** called the **MHC molecules** as well as genes coding for other proteins involved in host defence. MHC molecules were originally identified as the principal determinants of transplantation rejection. Later, their importance in immune responses was found to depend on the requirement for MHC molecules in the recognition of antigens by T cells. The fact that a given T cell will recognize antigen only when bound and presented by a particular MHC molecule is known as **MHC restriction**, or MHC-restricted antigen recognition **(40)**. Cells expressing MHC molecules are thus vital in activating the acquired immune response.

The human MHC is located on chromosome six and the group of genes that encodes cell surface antigen-presenting proteins is called the **human leukocyte antigen** system or HLA. There are two different groups of MHC genes involved in antigen presentation. These gene products are called **MHC class I** and **MHC class II** molecules. MHC class I molecules are encoded by genes named HLA-A, HLA-B and HLA-C. There are also three pairs of MHC class II genes named HLA-DR, HLA-DP and HLA-DQ. Most individuals are **heterozygous** at the level of the MHC loci. MHC genes are **expressed co-dominantly** meaning each individual expresses six different class I molecules (three from each copy of chromosome six). The HLA-DR gene cluster can contain extra genes, which means that there are more possibilities for class II molecules. The particular combination of MHC genes present on one chromosome is known as the **MHC haplotype**. As each MHC molecule can potentially present many different peptides to T cells, the presence of different MHC genes enables presentation of a much broader peptide range.

T cells can be classed into two groups distinguished by expression of the surface proteins CD4 and CD8, and accordingly in the class of MHC molecule recognized. MHC class I molecules are found on all nucleated cells and present endogenous antigens to CD8 T cells. MHC class II molecules are limited to immune cells, such as dendritic cells, macrophages and B cells. They present antigen of exogenous origin to CD4 T cells.

An additional group within the MHC can be classified as **MHC class III** genes. These encode a diverse group of molecules not involved in antigen presentation to T cells. MHC class III genes include genes for complement proteins and inflammatory cytokines, such as tumour necrosis factor (TNF) **(43)**.

Answers

40. See explanation
41. 1 – I; 2 – B; 3 – C, E, G; 4 – F; 5 – D; 6 – I; 7 – H
42. A – Nucleated cells, B – CD8, C – immune cells, D – CD4
43. Complement and cytokines

44. Fill in the blanks in the following sentences using options from the list below (each option can be used once, more than once or not at all)

Options

A. Four

B. α

C. Polymorphic

D. β$_2$-Microglobulin

E. II

F. I

G. γ

H. Five

1. MHC molecules consist of _____ extracellular protein domains
2. In MHC class I molecules, the _____ chain is longer than the _____ chain
3. In MHC class _____ molecules, both chains cross the membrane
4. The peptide-binding grooves of MHC molecules are highly _____

45. Label the following diagrams showing the structure of major histocompatibility complex molecules

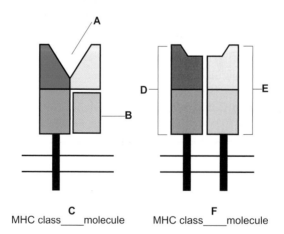

MHC class____molecule   MHC class____molecule

46. State why major histocompatibility complex class II molecules can accommodate longer peptides than major histocompatibility complex class I molecules

MHC, major histocompatibility complex

EXPLANATION: STRUCTURE OF MAJOR HISTOCOMPATIBILITY COMPLEX MOLECULES

Major histocompatibility complex (MHC) class I and MHC class II molecules have a similar overall structure consisting of **four extracellular protein domains**. In both cases, the two domains furthest from the membrane fold to create a **peptide-binding groove**.

MHC class I molecules consist of two polypeptide chains – the larger is designated as α and the smaller non-MHC-encoded chain is named β_2-microglobulin (β_2m). Only the α-chain crosses the membrane. For MHC class II molecules, the chains are designated α and β. Encoded in the MHC, both chains are of a similar size and have transmembrane portions (see figure).

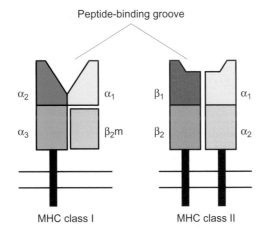

The peptide-binding grooves of both molecules are highly **polymorphic**. The resulting variations in the surface of the groove means a variety of peptides can be presented by different MHC molecules. The groove of the MHC class II molecule is more open than that of the class I molecule, enabling it to accommodate longer peptides **(46)**.

Answers

44. 1 – A; 2 – B, D; 3 – E; 4 – C
45. A – Peptide-binding groove, B – β_2-microglobulin, C – I, D – β-chain, E – α-chain, F – II
46. See explanation

47. What is antigen processing?

48. Considering major histocompatibility complex class I antigen processing

    a. MHC class I molecules usually present peptide fragments derived from extracellular proteins
    b. The proteasome is involved in MHC class I antigen processing
    c. IFN-γ increases proteasome efficiency
    d. TAP1 and TAP2 are involved in MHC class I antigen processing
    e. TAP1 and TAP2 are ATP-independent

49. Answer the following questions about major histocompatibility complex class I antigen processing

    a. State the origin of the peptide fragments presented by MHC class I molecules
    b. What is the proteasome?
    c. What is the role of the proteasome in MHC class I antigen processing?
    d. What is the role of the TAP molecules in MHC class I antigen processing?
    e. Where does the MHC class I molecule first associate with its peptide fragment?

50. Put the following statements about major histocompatibility complex class I antigen processing in the correct order

    a. Peptides are translocated into the endoplasmic reticulum via TAP
    b. Endogenous antigen is degraded by the proteasome
    c. Peptide:MHC complexes move to the cell surface
    d. Peptides associate with MHC class I molecules

ATP, adenosine triphosphate; ER, endoplasmic reticulum; IFN, interferon; MHC, major histocompatibility complex; TAP, transporter associated with antigen processing

EXPLANATION: ANTIGEN PROCESSING AND PRESENTATION I

As previously mentioned, T cells only recognize pathogen peptide fragments in conjunction with major histocompatibility complex (MHC) molecules. The generation of these fragments from a whole antigen is referred to as antigen processing **(47)**. The pathways involved in antigen processing differ between MHC class I and MHC class II molecules.

MHC class I antigen processing: MHC class I molecules typically present peptide fragments derived from **cytosolic** or **nuclear** (**endogenous**) proteins to **CD8** T cells. These fragments will normally originate from self-proteins, but are mainly of microbial origin during infection (A). The first stage involves **degradation** of the protein into smaller peptides by a multi-subunit proteolytic complex called the **proteasome** (B). Proteasome function becomes more efficient in the presence of interferon-γ (IFN-γ), a cytokine produced during many infections. The peptides are then **translocated** into the lumen of the membrane-bound **endoplasmic reticulum** (ER) of the cell. This is achieved via two ATP-dependent proteins named **TAP1** and **TAP2** (transporters associated with antigen processing; C). In the ER, the newly synthesized MHC class I molecules associate with specific peptide fragments determined by the residues in the peptide-binding groove (D). The complex then leaves the ER and moves to the **cell surface**.

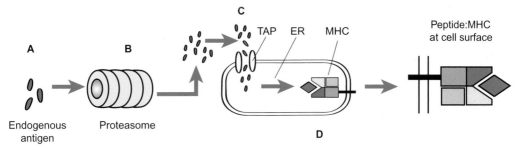

This processing pathway is particularly important during **viral infections** when viral proteins are present in the cytoplasm and nucleus. It enables presentation of viral antigens by cell surface MHC class I molecules, which then alerts cytotoxic CD8 T cells to the presence of infection.

Answers

47. See explanation
48. F T T T F
49. a – Endogenous (microbial or self), b – A multi-subunit proteolytic complex, c – It degrades intracellular proteins, d – They translocate peptides into the endoplasmic reticulum, e – Within the endoplasmic reticulum
50. b, a, d, c

51. **Fill in the blanks in the following statements concerning antigen processing and presentation using the options below (each option can be used once, more than once or not at all)**

Options

A. Endocytosis
B. Intracellular
C. Proteases
D. Exogenous
E. Exocytosis

F. Proteasome
G. Cathepsin L
H. Invariant chain
I. Cathepsin S
J. Amylase

1. MHC class II molecules usually present peptides of _____ origin
2. Antigen is taken up by a process called _____
3. Antigen held in vesicles is degraded by a group of enzymes known as _____
4. Examples of these enzymes include _____ and _____
5. The MHC molecule does not bind to peptide in the endoplasmic reticulum owing to the presence of the _____

52. **Answer the following questions about major histocompatibility complex class II antigen processing**

a. How are extracellular peptides stored after endocytosis?
b. How are the proteases that degrade endocytosed antigen activated?
c. Where is the MHC class II molecule itself assembled?
d. When is the invariant chain degraded?

ER, endoplasmic reticulum; Ii, invariant chain; MHC, major histocompatibility complex; MIIC, MHC class II compartment

EXPLANATION: ANTIGEN PROCESSING AND PRESENTATION II

Major histocompatibility complex (MHC class II) molecules typically present peptides of **exogenous** (or extracellular) origin that have been taken up into the cells via **endocytic vesicles (A)**. After endocytosis of an antigen, the endocytic vesicle becomes increasingly acidic, which activates various acid **proteases** that degrade the antigen **(B)**. The proteases thought to be involved include **cathepsin L** and **cathepsin S**. The MHC class II molecule is assembled in the endoplasmic reticulum (ER), as is the MHC class I molecule **(C)**. However, the presence of a protein known as the **invariant chain (Ii)**, which lies across the MHC molecule peptide-binding groove, prevents any peptides present in the ER from binding to MHC class II molecules at this site. Instead, the MHC class II molecules are directed into vesicles forming part of the **endosomal** pathway. These vesicles fuse with the endosomes containing the degraded antigenic peptide **(D)**. The Ii chain is then degraded, which frees the MHC peptide-binding groove for occupancy by peptide **(E)**. This is thought to occur in a particular endosomal compartment for peptide loading called the MIIC (MHC class II compartment). Following binding, the complex is then delivered to the cell surface **(F)**.

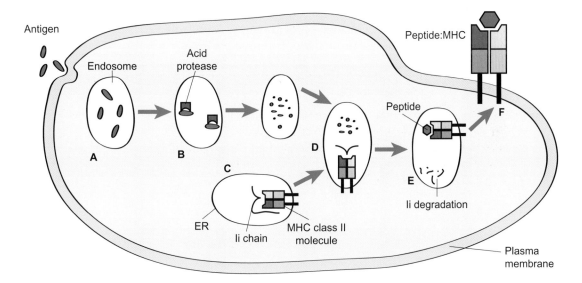

Antigen

Acid protease

Endosome

Peptide:MHC

Peptide

A

B

D

F

C

E

Ii degradation

ER

Ii chain

MHC class II molecule

Plasma membrane

Answers

51. 1 – D; 2 – A; 3 – C; 4 – G, I; 5 – H
52. a – In endocytic vesicles, b – By increasing acidity within the vesicle, c – Within the endoplasmic reticulum, d – Following fusion with the endocytic vesicle containing antigen

³

53. Regarding the structure of T cell receptors

a. The TCRs expressed by a single T cell are all identical
b. Most TCRs are composed of an α- and a β-chain
c. The variable region of each chain contains three binding loops called CDRs
d. TCR chains do not have a transmembrane region
e. The variable domain of the TCR chains contain the regions that bind the peptide: MHC complex
f. CDR3 interacts with peptide

54. Answer the following questions concerning T cell signalling

a. Name the amino acid sequences involved in initiation of the T cell signalling cascade
b. Where are these sequences located?

APC; activated antigen presenting cell; CDR, complementarity determining region; ITAM, immunoreceptor tyrosine-based activation motif; MHC, major histocompatibility complex; TCR, T cell receptor

EXPLANATION: T CELL RECEPTORS AND ANTIGEN RECOGNITION

Each T cell expresses about **30 000 identical antigen receptors** on its surface. Each chain can be divided into a **constant** region and a **variable** region. The T cell receptor (TCR) binds its complementary peptide: major histocompatability complex (MHC) complex via its variable regions. The variable region of each chain contains three binding loops, named **CDR1, CDR2** and **CDR3**. CDR1 and 2 bind mainly to the MHC molecule itself, whereas the CDR3 loops meet over the central amino acids of the peptide. Reflecting the large diversity in amino-acid sequences of the presented peptide, the CDR3 is the most **variable** loop.

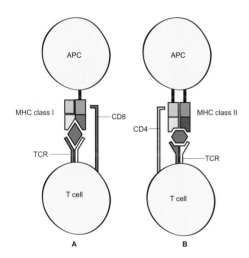

For a more efficient response, further binding between T cell **co-receptors** and the MHC molecule is required. CD8 is expressed on cytotoxic T cells and binds MHC class I molecules (A). CD4 is expressed on T-helper cells and binds MHC class II molecules (B). Thus, the need for co-receptor binding explains MHC molecule specificity for CD or CD8.

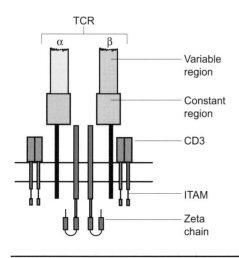

Upon TCR and co-receptor binding to the peptide:MHC complex presented by an activated antigen presenting cell (APC), the T cell itself is activated. This results from a **cascade** of signals leading to the activation of nuclear transcription factors, which **modulate expression** of different genes. Initiation of the signalling cascade involves amino-acid sequences called **immunoreceptor tyrosine-based activation motifs** or ITAMs. The TCR heterodimer of α- and β-chains binds antigen but cannot activate the T cell by itself, as it does not contain ITAMs. Instead, activation signals are produced by ITAM-containing signalling proteins that include a homodimer called the zeta chain and a complex called **CD3** found in close association with the TCR.

Answers
53. T T T F T T
54. a – ITAMs, b – CD3 and the zeta chains

55. **What antigen-presenting cell type is vital in the activation of nearly all T cell responses?**

56. **Put the following statements in relation to T cell activation in the correct order**

   a. T cell interaction with dendritic cell
   b. Phagocytosis of pathogen by dendritic cell
   c. Migration of dendritic cell to lymphoid tissue
   d. Activation of dendritic cell

57. **Describe some surface molecule changes seen when immature dendritic cells become activated**

58. **Fill in the blanks in the following paragraph relating to naive T cell migration using the options below (each option can be used once, more than once or not at all)**

Options

A. HEVs
B. Naive T cells
C. Capillary walls
D. Chemokine

E. Integrins
F. Smooth muscle cells
G. ICAM-2
H. LFA

Naive T cells enter lymphoid tissue by crossing _____. Migration is initiated by a _____ called CCL21, which binds CCR7 expressed by _____. This is followed by activation of _____, which act to arrest T cell movement. Within the lymphoid tissue, initial binding of a T cell with a dendritic cell is mediated by adhesion molecules, such as dendritic cell ICAM1 and _____, and T cell LFA

APC, antigen-presenting cell; HEV, high endothelial venuule; ICAM, intracellular adhesion molecule; LFA-1, leukocyte function-associated antigen; MHC, major histocompatibility complex

EXPLANATION: INITIATION OF THE ACQUIRED IMMUNE RESPONSE

An effective immune response is dependent on the coordinated action of both innate and acquired defences. Acquired defences are generally initiated by components of the innate response.

The cornerstone of initiation of the acquired immune response is naive T cell activation upon recognition of a specific peptide:MHC complex on the surface of an activated antigen-presenting cell (APC). Potent APCs named **dendritic cells** are thought to initiate nearly all *in vivo* T cell responses.

Immature dendritic cells, such as Langerhans cells found in the skin, **phagocytose** antigen at the site of infection via similar mechanisms to macrophages. They also have the ability to ingest surrounding fluid by a process called **macropinocytosis**. Following pathogen uptake, they become activated. This is typified by the expression of new peptide:MHC molecules as well as the upregulation of surface co-stimulatory molecules, such as CD80 and CD86 **(57)**. The activated dendritic cell then migrates to local lymphoid tissues. This is promoted by the following of chemokine gradients in a process known as **chemotaxis**. Langerhans cells, for example, move to nearby lymph nodes.

Meanwhile, naive T cells enter the lymph nodes by crossing special vessels named **high endothelial venules** (HEVs). Migration is thought to be mediated mainly by the chemokine **CCL21**, which is expressed by HEV endothelial cells and dendritic cells located in the lymphoid tissue. CCL21 binds the receptor **CCR7** expressed by naive T cells. Binding activates **integrins,** such as intracellular adhesion molecules (ICAMs) ICAM-1 and ICAM-2 on the endothelial surface, which act to arrest T cell movement along the HEV and allow movement into the lymphoid tissue.

Within the lymphoid tissue, initial interaction between naive T cells and dendritic cells involves cell-adhesion molecules, such as **ICAM-1, ICAM-2** (expressed on APCs as well as HEV endothelium) and **LFA-1** (the corresponding receptor on the T cell). The transient binding allows T cell **sampling** of the dendritic cell peptide:MHC complexes and possibly leads to T cell activation.

Answers

55. Dendritic cell
56. b, d, c, a
57. See explanation
58. A, D, B, E, G

59. **Label the following diagram of a typical T cell response**

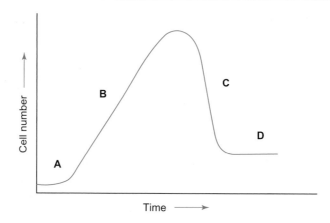

60. **Answer the following questions**

    a. What two signals do T cells require for activation?
    b. Name two co-stimulatory molecules seen on antigen-presenting cells and their corresponding T cell receptor
    c. What cytokine induces T cell proliferation? How does it act?
    d. What is programmed cell death also known as?
    e. Name two mechanisms of apoptosis that may occur during the contraction phase
    f. What are cells that survive the contraction phase called?

AICD, activation-induced cell death; APC, antigen-presenting cell; Il, interleukin; MHC, major histocompatibility complex

EXPLANATION: T CELL RESPONSES

The T cell response typically involves the following stages: activation; expansion; contraction; and memory formation.

Activation of naive T cells occurs in secondary lymphoid tissues and involves two signals. The first is the specific recognition of antigen bound to major histocompatability complex (MHC) molecules on the surface of a dendritic cell. The second signal also originates from this antigen-presenting cell (APC) and is termed **co-stimulation**.

Peptides derived from the invading microorganism will be bound by MHC molecules and presented on the surface of the dendritic cells (first signal). Cytokines, produced by the innate immune system in response to the infection and tissue damage, activate dendritic cells to express specific surface molecules, such as **CD80** and **CD86**, also known as B7.1 and B7.2. These are co-stimulatory molecules that are recognized by the receptor **CD28** on the T cell (second signal). As both signals are required for T cell activation, the requirement for co-stimulation limits the possibility that cells are activated in the absence of infection. In fact, activation of a T cell in the absence of co-stimulation leads to a state of non-responsiveness in the cell termed **anergy**. Upon successful activation, cells acquire effector functions that will be discussed later.

Rapid **expansion** in cell numbers occurs concurrently with acquisition of effector function. This depends on synthesis of the cytokine **IL-2** by activated T cells. IL-2 binding triggers completion of the cell cycle and thus rapid T cell proliferation.

Contraction in cell numbers occurs when no more antigen is presented to specific T cells. This stage is due to programmed cell death, also known as **apoptosis**. Effector cells are highly susceptible to apoptosis via a mechanism known as activation-induced cell death (AICD) and also by limited availability of growth factors, such as cytokines. Some cells survive contraction.

T cells that survive the contraction stage form a **long-lasting memory cell pool**. Memory cells can exert a **rapid** and **efficient** response upon re-exposure to antigen in the future.

Answers

59. A – Activation, B – expansion, C – contraction, D – Memory formation
60. a – Antigen presentation and co-stimulation; b – CD80, CD86, CD28; c – IL-2, triggers cell cycle completion; d – Apoptosis; e – Activation-induced cell death, cytokine limitation; f – Memory cells

61. Name two lineages of T-helper cells

62. Describe how T-helper type 1 cells activate macrophages

63. Fill in the blanks in following table

Cytokine(s)	Origin (T_H1 or T_H2)	Function
IFN-γ	A	B
C	D	Promotes T cell proliferation
E	F	Eosinophilia
IL-13	G	H

64. Answer the following questions using the cytokines named below

Options

A. IFN-γ
B. IL-4

1. Promotes the development of T_H1 cells
2. Promotes the development of T_H2 cells
3. Helps defend against helminths
4. Helps defend against intracellular viruses
5. Inhibits T_H2 cell development
6. Inhibits T_H1 cell development
7. Helps to activate macrophages

IFN, interferon; IL, interleukin; MHC, major histocompatibility complex; T_H1, T-helper type 1; T_H2, T-helper type 2; TNF, tumour necrosis factor

EXPLANATION: CD4 T CELLS

Also known as **T-helper cells**, CD4 T cells are vital in orchestrating immune responses. Upon activation by peptide:MHC class II complexes, naive CD4 T cells undergo proliferation and differentiation into two different lineages designated **T-helper type 1 (T_H1)** and **T-helper type 2 (T_H2)**, each characterized by the production of different cytokines.

T_H1 cells produce high levels of **IFN-γ** and provide cell-mediated immunity against intracellular pathogens, such as *Leishmania* species and mycobacteria. An important role of T_H1 cells is the **activation of macrophages**. Bacterial components such as lipopolysaccharide have been shown to sensitize macrophages to activation by IFN-γ but, in many cases, activation requires T_H1 cells expressing a surface molecule called CD40 ligand (CD40L) to bind the macrophage receptor CD40 **(62)**. In addition, activated T_H1 cells are an important source of IFN-γ itself. Activated macrophages then destroy intracellular pathogens. T_H1 cells also produce cytokines, such as tumour necrosis factor (**TNF**), which is required for an effective inflammatory response, and **IL-2**, which promotes T cell proliferation.

T_H2 cells produce cytokines, such as **IL-4, IL-10, IL-13 and IL-5**, and help with immunity against extracellular pathogens including helminths. The T_H2 cytokines promote immune defences including eosinophilia (IL-5), fibrosis (IL-13, IL-10), mucus secretion and smooth muscle contraction.

Helper T cells are also vital in promoting the development of B cell-mediated humoral responses. This will be explained in more detail later.

An important factor influencing the lineage choice of T_H1 or T_H2 is the surrounding **cytokine environment**. IFN-γ promotes the production of T_H1 cells. These in turn secrete high levels of IFN-γ, thus amplifying an effective response against intracellular pathogens and inhibiting T_H2 cell development. In a similar way, IL-4 promotes the production of T_H2 cells.

Answers

61. T_H1 and T_H2
62. See explanation
63. A – T_H1, B – Macrophage activation/antiviral, C – IL-2, D – T_H1, E – IL-5, F – T_H2, G – T_H2, H – Fibrosis
64. 1 – A, 2 – B, 3 – B, 4 – A, 5 – A, 6 – B, 7 – A

65. Regarding CD8 T cells

a. CD8 T cells are also known as helper T cells
b. CD8 T cells are also known as cytotoxic T cells
c. Naive CD8 T cells direct from the thymus can lyse target cells
d. Two signals are required for naive CD8 T cell activation
e. Recognition of antigen bound to MHC class I molecules is one of the signals required for naive CD8 T cell activation

66. Fill in the blanks in the following statements concerning CD8 T cells using the options below (each option can be used once, more than once or not at all)

Options

A. Viruses
B. Co-stimulation
C. B
D. IFN-γ
E. Perforin
F. Dendritic
G. Fas
H. Activation

I. Tumours
J. Granzymes
K. CD4 T
L. TNF
M. Caspases
N. IL-5
O. IL-2

1. Dendritic cells can provide the two signals required for cytotoxic T cell activation against _____ but generally not against _____
2. In the response to a viral infection, _____ cells and _____ cells are usually required for cytotoxic T cell activation
3. In the response to a viral infection, CD4 T cells induce strong _____ for cytotoxic T cells and secrete cytokines such as _____, which induces proliferation
4. Cytotoxic T cells kill by the release of _____ and _____, which together induce apoptosis
5. Activated cytotoxic T cells can express a surface molecule called Fas ligand, which binds _____ and activates apoptotic enzymes called _____
6. Activated cytotoxic T cells can secrete cytokines including _____ and _____

CTL, cytotoxic T lymphocyte; IFN, interferon; IL, interleukin; MHC, major histocompatibility complex; NK, natural killer; TNF, tumour necrosis factor

EXPLANATION: CD8 T CELLS

CD8 T cells, also known as **cytotoxic T lymphocytes** (CTLs), are vital in clearing **viral** infection and also play a role in controlling tumour cells. Upon exit from the thymus, naive CTLs cannot lyse target cells. Functional activation requires two signals: first, the **recognition of antigen** bound to MHC class I molecules; and second, strong **co-stimulation**. Mature dendritic cells can provide both signals in responses against some tumours. However, in viral infections, the additional presence of CD4 T cells seems to be required to induce sufficiently strong co-stimulation and secrete some required cytokines, such as IL-2.

Activated CTLs recognize and kill upon recognition of specific antigen on the surface of a target cell. In common with natural killer (NK) cells, CTLs can release **perforin** and **granzymes**, which results in death of the target cell by **apoptosis**. However, activated CTLs also express a surface molecule called **Fas** ligand. This binds the molecule Fas on a target cell membrane and activates caspases, which induce apoptosis.

CTLs can also secrete some cytokines including: **IFN-γ,** which promotes an antiviral environment by activating macrophages and increasing expression of **peptide:MHC**. CTLs also secrete **TNF**, which promotes inflammation.

Answers

65. F T F T T
66. 1 – I, A; 2 – F, K; 3 – B, O; 4 – E, J; 5 – G, M; 6 – D, L

67. In T cell–B cell interactions, what is meant by linked recognition?

68. Put the following statements about T cell–B cell interactions in the order in which events take place

   a. T cell upregulates CD40L and produces cytokines
   b. T cell activated
   c. T cell recognizes antigen presented by B cell
   d. Isotype switching
   e. B cell proliferates
   f. Dendritic cell processes and presents antigen
   g. B cell differentiates into plasma cell

69. Concerning T cell–B cell interactions

   a. Antibody isotype switching requires T cell help
   b. CD40–CD40L interaction is not important in interactions between T and B cells
   c. T_H1 cells are better than T_H2 cells at promoting B cell responses.
   d. The cytokine IL-13 promotes formation of IgE
   e. T cell help is not required in the formation of germinal centres

---

Ig, immunoglobulin; IL, interleukin; MHC, major histocompatibility complex; mRNA, messenger ribonucleic acid; T_H1, T-helper type 1; T_H2, T-helper type 2

EXPLANATION: T CELL–B CELL INTERACTIONS

In common with T cells, B cell activation requires two signals. The first is via the **B cell antigen receptor**, and the second involves **accessory signals**. The accessory signal can originate from the antigen itself, but usually the presence of an effector T-helper cell is required. For successful T cell–B cell interactions, both cells must respond to the same antigen in what is called **linked recognition (67)**.

The naive T cell is first activated following the recognition of peptide:MHC on the surface of an activated dendritic cell in a lymph node. Once activated, it can then bind the identical peptide:MHC displayed on the surface of an antigen-presenting B cell. The activated T cell expresses the surface molecule **CD40 ligand**, which binds to **CD40** on the B cell. This interaction drives the B cell into the cell cycle, and feeds back to promote T cell secretion of cytokines. **IL-4**, produced by effector T_H2 cells when they recognize specific peptide:MHC on the surface of a B cell, is thought to enhance B cell proliferation. After several rounds of division, B cells **differentiate** into antibody-secreting plasma cells.

Switching between different antibody isotypes is also dependent on T-helper cells, as **CD40L–CD40 interaction** and secretion of different **cytokines** are both required. Cytokines contribute to isotype switching by stimulating the formation and splicing of mRNA transcribed from switch recombination sites that lie on the genome near the constant region of the heavy-chain immunoglobulin. T_H1 cells are relatively poor inducers of isotype switching compared to T_H2 cells, reflecting their role in responses to intracellular pathogens rather than humoral immunity. Different cytokines preferentially promote different antibody isotypes. For example, the T_H2 cytokine IL-13 stimulates switching to IgE production. IgE contributes to T_H2-mediated responses to extracellular pathogens.

T-helper cells are also required for further stages in B cell responses, including **affinity maturation** and the formation of **germinal centres**.

Answers

67. See explanation
68. f, b, c, a, e, g, d
69. T F F T F

70. Explain why secondary lymphoid tissues are important in an immune response

71. Fill in the blanks in the following statements concerning lymphocyte recirculation using the options below (each option can be used once, more than once or not at all)

Options

A. CCL21 C. CXCR5
B. CCR7 D. CXCL13

1. The chemokine _____ is important in the extravasation of lymphocytes into lymph nodes
2. The chemokine _____ is secreted by dendritic cells and HEV cells
3. Naive B cells express high levels of the receptor _____, which potentiates follicular migration
4. Follicular dendritic cells secrete high levels of the chemokine _____
5. Naive T cells express high levels of the receptor _____, which means they remain within the cortical areas

72. Considering cellular migration within a lymph node

a. B cells cannot move into T cell areas
b. T cells cannot move into B cell areas
c. B cells can encounter antigen in a variety of areas
d. Naive T cells do not express the cell surface receptor CCR7
e. Activated T cells can express the cell surface receptor CXCR5

HEV, high endothelial venule; MHC, major histocompatibility complex

EXPLANATION: LYMPHOCYTE RECIRCULATION

As mentioned previously, initiation of an adaptive immune response occurs within specialized secondary lymphoid tissues, such as the lymph nodes and spleen. Thus, the primary function of secondary lymphoid organs is to allow antigen-presenting cells, and antigen-specific B and T cells to come into close contact **(70)**. The movement of lymphocytes and dendritic cells both into and within secondary lymphoid organs depends on different gradients of mediators called **chemokines**.

Initially, chemokines contribute to the **extravasation** of lymphocytes and dendritic cells from high endothelial venules (HEVs) into the lymph nodes. As mentioned previously, this is mediated mainly by the chemokine CCL21. Once the cells have entered the lymph nodes, they undergo **compartmental homing** owing to differential chemokine expression.

T cells and dendritic cells remain in the cortical areas. The attraction of the naive T cells towards the waiting dendritic cells is mediated by maintenance of T cell expression of the surface receptor **CCR7**. This is bound by **CCL21**, which is secreted by dendritic cells as well as HEV cells. The T cells can then sample the dendritic cell peptide:MHC and possibly initiate an adaptive immune response.

B cells may first encounter antigen in several locations including the blood, the area around HEVs, and within follicles. The migratory pathway of the naive B cell is also dependent on chemokine expression. For example, B cells express high levels of the receptor **CXCR5** specific for the chemokine **CXCL13**. CXCL13 is secreted by follicular dendritic cells, which are located in the follicles and are crucially involved in long-term B cell antibody responses. Upon encountering antigen, B cells **upregulate chemokine receptors**, which promote migration to T cell areas and **potentiate efficient interaction** between the two cell types. Correspondingly, some activated T cells can upregulate receptors, such as CXCR5, and move into B cell follicles. Here, they can provide help for B cells in the processes of antibody isotype switching and affinity maturation.

Thus, migration through a secondary lymphoid organ is optimized to allow successful interaction of the different cell types and the production of an efficient immune response.

Answers

70. See explanation
71. 1 – A, 2 – A, 3 – C, 4 – D, 5 – B
72. F F T F T

73. What is immunological tolerance? What may breakdown of immune tolerance cause?

74. Fill in the blanks in the following paragraph concerning tolerance using the options below (each option can be used once, more than once or not at all)

Options

A. B cells
B. Negative
C. Avidity
D. Macrophages

E. Apoptosis
F. Positive
G. Thymus
H. Periphery

Central tolerance occurs in the _____. It involves _____ selection, where self-reactive T cells are deleted by _____. It is mediated by antigen-presenting cells, such as dendritic cells and _____. Susceptibility of T cells to this process is thought to depend on a threshold of _____

75. Answer the following questions about central tolerance

a. Thymic epithelial cells express a transcription factor called AIRE. What does it do?
b. Transgenic mice lacking AIRE are born. What type of disease do they develop?

MHC, major histocompatibility complex; TCR, T cell receptor

EXPLANATION: T CELL TOLERANCE I

Immunological tolerance refers to the ability of the host to **avoid self-reactive** and **potentially damaging immune responses (73)**. Tolerance relates to a fundamental and hotly debated paradigm of immunology – the discrimination between 'self' and 'non-self'. Correct recognition of immunological self should lead to central and peripheral immune tolerance, whereby there is no immune response, or only an attenuated one, against the body's own normal components. Breakdown of immune tolerance may lead to **autoimmunity (73)**.

Central tolerance occurs in the **thymus**, the site of T cell development. In the thymus, **positive selection** initially acts to ensure formation of a T cell repertoire with inherent specificity for MHC molecules. This is required for optimal recognition of MHC-bound foreign antigens. Next, **negative selection** involves the **apoptotic deletion** of thymocytes that interact with MHC-bound self-peptides at a very high affinity. Strongly self-reactive cells are potentially harmful, if activated in the periphery, and may initiate autoimmune damage. If completely effective, negative selection would purge the T cell repertoire of self-reactive T cells. Thus, it forms the basis of central tolerance.

Several different T cell types mediate negative selection in the thymus. The most important are professional **antigen-presenting cells** derived from the bone marrow, such as **dendritic cells** and **macrophages**. These cells induce tolerance in the repertoire by presenting self-peptide:MHC complexes to the developing thymocytes. However, an obvious problem is that many tissue-specific proteins found in the periphery would not be expected to be present in the thymus. This raises the possibility that cells reactive for a self-antigen that are absent from the thymus may avoid negative selection. Potentially, they could exit into the periphery and cause autoimmune damage. However, a subset of thymic epithelial cells minimize the chance of this occurring by upregulating expression of a **transcription factor** called **AIRE**. AIRE promotes promiscuous gene expression, and maximizes the variety of self-peptides presented to the developing thymocytes **(75a)**. Thus, lack of AIRE would lead to widespread autoimmune disease **(75b)**.

Murine studies have suggested susceptibility of T cells to negative selection depends on a **threshold of receptor avidity**, above which deletion occurs. This in turn relates to variables including T cell receptor (TCR) or co-receptor expression, antigen density and TCR affinity for the peptide:MHC complex.

Answers

73. See explanation
74. G, B, E, D, C
75. a – See explanation, b – Diffuse autoimmune disease

76. With regard to peripheral tolerance

a. Peripheral tolerance occurs in the thymus
b. Peripheral tuning involves an increase in T cell sensitivity as the T cells remain in the periphery
c. Anergy is a state of heightened responsiveness
d. Anergic T cells result from TCR stimulation in the absence of inflammation

77. What is the name given to the mechanism of cell death following continuous activation? Name two occasions when this mechanism may be useful

78. Answer the following questions

a. What is the function of regulatory T cells?
b. Where do these cells originate?
c. What two markers do they characteristically express?
d. Name a secreted cytokine vital for their inhibitory function
e. Name two inhibitory effects of IL-10

AICD, activation-induced cell death; IL, interleukin; TCR, T cell receptor; T_H1, T-helper type 1

EXPLANATION: T CELL TOLERANCE II

Immune tolerance in the periphery comes into play particularly upon the failure of central tolerance mechanisms to purge the T cell repertoire of autoreactivity. There are numerous possible mechanisms to explain peripheral tolerance.

For example, it has been suggested that the reactivity of T cells circulating in the periphery is modified by continual interactions with self-peptide and that, consequently, the cells **decrease in sensitivity** over time. This idea of **peripheral tuning** has been supported by evidence from transgenic mice. **Anergy** is a state of non-responsiveness where the cell fails to respond to its specific antigen. It has been proposed that cells become anergic when stimulated through their TCR in the absence of other co-stimulatory signals indicating the presence of inflammation, e.g. absence of CD80 and CD86 on the surface of the dendritic cell. Thus, anergy will limit T cell activation by a self-antigen in the absence of infection.

Another mechanism called **activation-induced cell death** (AICD) also exists. This occurs in cells that have undergone a period of excessive activation. It is vital in limiting the numbers of immune cells following clearance of infection, but may also have a role in deleting cells that are continuously activated by self-antigen **(77)**.

An additional peripheral tolerance mechanism involves a subset of **regulatory T cells** that actively downregulate the proliferation and activation of self-reactive T cells **(78a)**. These cells originate from the thymus and express high levels of the surface molecule **CD25** as well as **CD4**. They secrete the cytokine **IL-10**, which is thought to be important in mediating their inhibitory action. IL-10 inhibits both the ability of dendritic cells to activate T cells and the differentiation of T_H1 cells **(78e)**.

Answers

76. F F F T
77. Activation-induced cell death (AICD), See explanation
78. a – See explanation, b – Thymus, c – CD25 and CD4, d – IL-10, e – See explanation

79. Concerning B cell tolerance

a. B cell tolerance is achieved by testing B cell reactivity to self-molecules in the bone marrow
b. Receptor editing involves genetic rearrangement of the immunoglobulin heavy chain
c. Receptor editing can change a self-reactive cell to a cell with no self-reaction
d. A persistently self-reactive cell that has experienced exhaustive receptor editing may undergo apoptosis in the bone marrow
e. A cell with no self-reactivity can leave the bone marrow for the periphery

80. Fill in the blanks in the following paragraph concerning B cell tolerance using the options below (each option can be used once, more than once or not at all)

Options

A. Little
B. Can
C. Blocked
D. Considerable

E. Anergic
F. Stimulated
G. Cannot

B cells that encounter soluble self-antigen may become _____. These cells express _____ surface immunoglobulin. Their signalling pathways involved in activation are _____. The cells _____ be activated

81. What term refers to B cells in the periphery that remain unaware of their self-antigen? Name two mechanisms by which this may occur

Ig, immunoglobulin

EXPLANATION: B CELL TOLERANCE

The requirement for B cell tolerance is possibly not as vital as T cell tolerance because B cells require T cell help for optimal responses to most antigens. Nevertheless, B cells also undergo central tolerance mechanisms in the **bone marrow** and peripheral tolerance mechanisms elsewhere in the body.

As discussed previously, B cells develop in the bone marrow. Following formation of immature B cells, the cells are tested for their ability to bind self-molecules. Cells that bind a self-antigen strongly can be rescued from apoptosis by further genetic rearrangement of their light chain to give new receptor specificity. This process is termed **receptor editing**. If receptor editing is successful, the cell expresses membrane-bound IgM and IgD, and can leave for the periphery. If exhaustive light-chain rearrangements continue to give a self-reactive cell, the cell will undergo **apoptosis**.

In the periphery, mature B cells become **inactivated** if they encounter soluble self-antigen in the absence of T cell help. Thus, effective T cell tolerance has an important role in maintaining B cell tolerance. The inactive B cells are in a state of **anergy**. They express very little surface immunoglobulin and appear to have a block in the signalling pathways needed for their activation. Once a B cell is anergic, it cannot be activated by specific antigen, even with help from specific T cells. There is also evidence that mature B cells can undergo direct apoptosis if they encounter larger multivalent antigens in the periphery.

A final fate for self-reactive B cells in the periphery is termed **ignorance**. Such cells remain immunologically 'ignorant' of their self-antigen. This may be due to very weak interaction between the antigen and B cell, which means that little intracellular signal is generated upon binding and the cell is not activated (81). Alternatively, anatomical distribution may mean the B cell never encounters the antigen, e.g. the antigen is sequestered within the brain (81).

Answers

79. T F T T T
80. E, A, C, G
81. Ignorance, See explanation

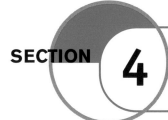

IMMUNE RESPONSES TO INFECTION

IMMUNE RESPONSES TO INFECTION

---

1. With regard to responses to extracellular bacterial infection

    a. *Streptococci* are extracellular bacterial pathogens
    b. Gram-negative cocci are never found extracellularly
    c. Extracellular bacteria can produce toxins
    d. Extracellular bacteria never induce inflammation
    e. An inflammatory response is always beneficial to the host

---

2. Fill in the blanks in the following paragraph concerning innate immune responses to extracellular bacteria using the options below (each option can be used once, more than once or not at all)

Options

    A. TNF   **F.** Monocytes
    B. Shock   **G.** IL-2
    C. Neutrophils   **H.** Fibrinolysis
    D. IL-1   **I.** Macrophages
    E. Leukocytes   **J.** Complement

Extracellular bacteria can be phagocytosed by cells such as _____, _____ and _____.
These cells can produce cytokines including _____ and _____, which potentiate
inflammation and attract _____. Excessive cytokine release can lead to a systemic pathology
and potentially fatal _____. Activation of the _____ cascade is also important

---

3. Answer the following questions about adaptive immune responses to extracellular bacteria

    a. Which T cell subset is vital in controlling extracellular bacterial infection?
    b. How do these T cells act?
    c. How can extracellular bacteria directly stimulate B cell responses?

---

4. Describe the importance of IgG and IgM in responses to extracellular bacteria

---

Ig, immunoglobulin; IL, interleukin; MHC, major histocompatibility complex; TNF, tumour necrosis factor

EXPLANATION: RESPONSES TO EXTRACELLULAR BACTERIAL INFECTION

Extracellular bacteria include gram-positive pyogenic cocci, such as *Staphylococcus* and *Streptococcus* spp., as well as some gram-negative cocci and many gram-negative bacilli, including enteric *Escherichia coli*. Extracellular bacteria can cause **tissue destruction** by the production of various **toxins**, which may have cytotoxic activity and stimulate **inflammation**.

Innate immune mechanisms: A principal innate immune mechanism involved in protecting against extracellular bacterial infections is **phagocytosis** mediated by neutrophils, monocytes and macrophages. These activated cells then produce cytokines, such as **tumour necrosis factor** (**TNF**) and **interleukin-1** (**IL-1**), which potentiate inflammation and aid leukocyte recruitment. Resultant inflammatory injury of normal tissues is a side-effect of these pro-inflammatory cytokines. Excessive release of cytokines, primarily TNF, can lead to severe systemic inflammatory tissue damage and, ultimately, can result in septic shock, which may be fatal. **Complement** activation is also important in host defence when it acts to lyse microbes and promote inflammation.

Acquired immune mechanisms: The T cell response to extracellular bacteria depends on **CD4 T cells** activated by bacterial antigens presented by major histocompatibility complex (MHC) class II molecules. As explained previously, CD4 T cells can then function as helper cells to stimulate antibody production and improve macrophage killing of internalized pathogens **(3b)**. The antibodies produced, such as **immunoglobulin G** (**IgG**) and **IgM,** may have a role in opsonization, complement activation and toxin neutralization**(4)**. The polysaccharide cell walls or capsules of some extracellular pathogens may also be able to activate B cells directly and stimulate production of IgM **(3c)**.

Answers

1. T F T F F
2. C, F, I, A, D, E, B, J
3. a – CD4, b – See explanation, c – See explanation
4. See explanation

5. Describe the role of type 1 interferons in viral infections

6. Considering responses to viral infection

    a. Interferons reduce NK cell activity
    b. Activated NK cells can lyse virally infected cells
    c. Innate immune mechanisms can completely clear a viral infection
    d. Acquired immune mechanisms can completely clear a viral infection
    e. CD8 T cells are vital in eradicating viral infection
    f. CD8 T cells recognize antigen presented by MHC class I molecules
    g. Activated CD8 T cells can directly lyse virally infected cells
    h. Activated CD4 T cell can directly lyse virally infected cells

7. Why are CD4 T cells important in clearing viral infection?

8. Fill in the blanks in the following paragraph concerning intracellular bacteria using the options below (each option can be used once, more than once or not at all)

Options

A. Phagocytosis	**F.** IL-4
B. CD4	**G.** CD8
C. Class II	**H.** Class III
D. CD3	**I.** Class I
E. IFN-γ	**J.** Antibody

One of the principal immune mechanisms acting against bacteria is _____ by cells, such as macrophages. Activation of _____ T cells by bacterial antigen:MHC class II complexes leads to the production of cytokines, such as _____, which enhances macrophage killing of intracellular pathogens. _____T cells may also kill infected cells following recognition of bacterial antigens presented on surface MHC _____ molecules

IFN, interferon; IL, interleukin; MHC, major histocompatibility complex; NK, natural killer

EXPLANATION: RESPONSES TO INTRACELLULAR PATHOGENS

Viruses are obligate **intracellular** pathogens. They replicate within cells, often using the protein synthesis machinery of the host cell. A number of **bacteria** are also capable of surviving within host cells, e.g. *Mycobacterium tuberculosis*.

Innate immune mechanisms (viruses): Viral infection stimulates the production of type 1 **interferons** (IFN-α and IFN-β) by infected cells. These induce a state of **viral resistance** in surrounding cells and also enhance the action of **natural killer (NK) cells (5)**. Activated NK cells are very important in lysing infected cells. However, it has been demonstrated that innate mechanisms can only control a virus; acquired mechanisms are required to clear the infection.

Acquired immune mechanisms (viruses): Very early in infection, **antibodies** may be important in binding to viral envelopes or capsid proteins and preventing cellular invasion. However, the most important acquired immune mechanism is the action of **CD8 T cells**. CD8 T cells recognize virally infected cells by the presence of viral peptides displayed on the cell surface by MHC class I molecules. They can then **lyse** the infected cell via the combined action of perforin and granzymes. Co-stimulation and cytokines produced by CD4 T cells activated by any endogenous viral antigens are important in attaining a full CD8 T cell response **(7)**.

Immune mechanisms (intracellular bacteria): One of the principal immune mechanisms acting against bacteria is **phagocytosis**. However, many bacteria, so-called intracellular bacteria, are relatively resistant to phagocytic degradation and can actively replicate within phagosomes. In these cases, activation of **CD4 T cells** by bacterial antigen:MHC II complexes on the cell surface leads to the production of cytokines, such as **IFN-γ**. IFN-γ enhances macrophage phagocytosis and degradative function, thus enhancing bacterial killing. This often eradicates the intracellular pathogen. **CD8 T cells** may also kill infected cells following recognition of bacterial antigens presented on surface MHC class I molecules.

Answers

5. See explanation
6. F T F T T T T F
7. See explanation
8. A, B, E, G, I

9. Fill in the blanks in the following paragraph concerning malarial infection using the options below (each option can be used once, more than once or not at all)

Options

A. 1
B. Erythrocytes
C. Opsonization
D. Macrophages
E. IFN-γ
F. Lymphocytes

G. *Plasmodium*
H. Hepatocytes
I. 2
J. IL-1
K. *Cryptosporidium*
L. Cytotoxicity

A protozoan parasite called _____ causes malaria. Malarial infection induces a type _____ immune response. Free parasites can be phagocytosed by _____ expressing the receptor CD36. T-helper cells contribute by secreting the cytokine _____. Antibody binding may reduce parasite invasion of _____ and _____. Antibody can also promote phagocytosis through _____

10. Regarding responses to helminth infection

a. Helminth infection induces a type 2 immune response
b. The signature cytokine produced in a type 2 immune response is IFN-γ
c. Helminth infection is associated with strong IgE, eosinophil and mast cell responses
d. IL-4 can stimulate smooth muscle in the intestine
e. IL-4 and IL-13 are not useful in the expulsion of gastrointestinal nematodes

11. Answer the following questions about *Schistosoma* spp. infection

a. *Schistosoma* spp. infection is associated with very high levels of which antibody isotype?
b. Which type of immune response promotes switching to this antibody isotype?
c. Which cytokine promotes eosinophil production in the bone marrow?
d. Name the mechanism by which eosinophils then act to kill the organism

ADCC, antibody-dependent cell-mediated cytotoxicity; FC, fragment crystallizable; IFN, interferon; Ig, immunoglobulin; IL, interleukin; T_H1, T-helper type 1; T_H2, T-helper type 2

EXPLANATION: RESPONSES TO PARASITIC INFECTION

Parasitic infection refers mainly to infection with **protozoa** (unicellular organisms) and **helminths** (worms). Parasites vary greatly in their structure and biochemistry, and often elicit significantly different immune responses.

Protozoan infection: The most common protozoan infection is probably due to the *Plasmodium* parasite, which causes malaria. In malarial infection, as with other protozoa, an overall **T-helper type 1 (T_H1) immune response** is induced. The exact immune mechanisms seen in malaria are stage-specific and vary as the parasites are initially cleared from the circulation, then replicate within the liver, and finally escape to invade erythrocytes. For example, free parasites can be phagocytosed by **macrophages** that bind to parasitic surface antigens via a scavenger receptor called **CD36**. Following activation by innate antigen-presenting cells, T_H1 cells also help by secreting **IFN-γ**, which promotes macrophage action and intracellular killing. Additionally, **antibody action** is important in malarial infection. Antibody binding may reduce parasite invasion of **hepatocytes** and **erythrocytes**, and promote phagocytosis by opsonization.

Helminth infection: Acquired immune mechanisms are the cornerstone of immunity to helminths. Helminth infection induces a **type 2 immune response** characterized by T_H2 cells secreting significant quantities of cytokines including IL-4, IL-5, IL-9 and IL-13, and consequently the development of strong **IgE, eosinophil** and **mast cell responses**. An unanswered question relates to how the host is able to first recognize the presence of a helminth and then induce a T_H2 response. It is possible that recognition by unknown pattern recognition receptors leads to early production of IL-4. In the case of helminths found within the gastrointestinal tract, the ability to expel nematodes is closely linked to the extent of the T_H2 response. For example, in infection with the intestinal nematode *Trichinella spiralis*, **IL-4** and **IL-13** stimulate intestinal smooth muscle cell contraction, promoting peristaltic ejection of the worm, and **IL-13** stimulates mucus secretion, which inhibits worm attachment. As mentioned previously, T_H2 cytokines also promote antibody isotype switching to **IgE**.

Production of specific IgE is known to be particularly important in fighting infection by *Schistosoma* spp., which are helminths that live within the portal vasculature. Following IgE binding of the worm, **eosinophils** (bone marrow production of which is stimulated by the T_H2 cytokine **IL-5**) attach to the opsonized organism via high-affinity Fc receptors. The eosinophils then release cytotoxic mediators, such as peroxidase, and mediate **antibody-dependent cell-mediated cytotoxicity (ADCC)**.

Answers

9. G, A, D, E, B, H, C
10. T F T T F
11. a – IgE, b – Type 2, c – IL-5, d – Antibody-dependent cell-mediated cytotoxicity

CLINICAL IMMUNOLOGY

CLINICAL IMMUNOLOGY

1. Match the following options to the appropriate definition (each option can be used once, more than once or not at all)

Options

A. Hypersensitivity reaction
B. Allergy
C. Autoimmunity

1. A harmful immune response to an otherwise innocuous, non-microbial, exogenous antigen
2. Any inappropriate or excessive immune response that causes damage to one's own tissues
3. A harmful immune response directed against self-antigens resulting in damage to one's own tissue

2. Match the following options to the appropriate type of hypersensitivity reaction (each option can be used once, more than once or not at all)

Options

A. Type 1   C. Type 3
B. Type 2   D. Type 4

1. These are responsible for the majority of allergic reactions
2. These are mediated through formation of immune complexes
3. These are mediated through the binding of antibodies either directly to host antigens or exogenous antigens bound to host cells
4. This type of hypersensitivity reaction is also known as delayed-type hypersensitivity
5. The antigens involved in this type of hypersensitivity reaction are always soluble
6. The antibodies responsible for this type of hypersensitivity reaction are found primarily bound to the surface of mast cells
7. This type of hypersensitivity reaction is T cell mediated

IG, immunoglobulin; MHC, major histocompatibility complex

EXPLANATION: HYPERSENSITIVITY REACTIONS

The physiological role of the immune system is to protect the host from infection. However, excessive or unnecessary immune responses can cause considerable damage to one's own tissues. Such damaging responses are termed **hypersensitivity reactions**, and there are four main types of these, differentiated by the mechanisms involved. Types 1–3 are mediated through antibody, while type 4 reactions are cell-mediated. Hypersensitivity reactions include **allergies**, in which immune responses are induced against innocuous exogenous antigens, as well as **autoimmune diseases**, in which responses are inappropriately mounted against self-antigens.

Type 1: These are the **most common** form of hypersensitivity reactions and constitute most allergic reactions. They are mediated through specific binding of antigen to immunoglobulin E (IgE) bound to the surface of **mast cells**, resulting in the release of **inflammatory mediators**, including histamine.

Type 2: This type of hypersensitivity reaction is mediated by IgG or IgM antibodies that cause tissue damage by binding to antigens and **inducing host defence mechanisms**. Examples include certain **drug reactions**, which can occur if antibodies are formed against a drug that binds to host cells, resulting in targeting of the cell. Similar mechanisms are responsible for many autoimmune conditions, in which antibodies are formed that directly target self-antigens and are, therefore, known as **autoantibodies**.

Type 3: These responses are mediated by IgG antibodies directed against soluble antigens. When these antibodies bind antigen, they form antigen–antibody aggregates known as **immune complexes**. These complexes tend to be deposited in certain areas, such as the **blood vessels** and the **glomeruli** of the kidney, where they induce an inflammatory response resulting in tissue damage.

Type 4: These hypersensitivity reactions are **mediated by T cells**. They occur when exogenous antigens are taken up and processed by self-cells and displayed on the cell surface in conjunction with MHC molecules. The peptide:MHC complexes are then recognized by CD4 or CD8 T cells, which mount an immune response by either releasing inflammatory cytokines or killing the self-cell. The subsequent inflammatory response takes 24–48 hours to develop and, consequently, these reactions are also known as **delayed-type hypersensitivity** reactions.

Answers

1. 1 – B, 2 – A, 3 – C
2. 1 – A, 2 – C, 3 – B, 4 – D, 5 – C, 6 – A, 7 – D

3. Concerning the factors that contribute to development of type 1 hypersensitivity reactions

   a. T_H2 T cell responses are required to induce IgE production by B cells
   b. Antigen delivery by the mucosal route favours IgE production
   c. Most allergies develop to antigens we are exposed to in very high doses
   d. Small, highly soluble protein antigens often induce IgE response and, therefore, act as allergens
   e. All individuals are equally susceptible to developing allergic reactions

4. Fill in the blanks in the following paragraph regarding the immediate phase of allergic responses using the options below (each option can be used once, more than once or not at all)

Options

A. Anergy
B. Histamine
C. Mast cells
D. Inflammation

E. Degranulation
F. Contraction
G. Neutrophils
H. Proteases

Once produced, most IgE is found in the tissues bound to the surface of _____. When the IgE is cross-linked by antigen, the cell is induced to undergo _____. This results in the release of a number of inflammatory mediators, including _____ and _____. These have several immediate effects, including local _____, smooth muscle _____ and tissue destruction

5. With regard to the late phase of type 1 hypersensitivity reactions

   a. This usually occurs within an hour of exposure to antigen
   b. This is brought about by release of preformed inflammatory mediators stored within mast cell granules
   c. Eosinophils are recruited in the late-phase reaction
   d. T_H1 cells have an important role in promoting the further production of IgE during the late-phase reaction

Ig, immunoglobulin; T_H1, T-helper type 1; T_H2, T-helper type 2

EXPLANATION: TYPE 1 HYPERSENSITIVITY REACTIONS – MECHANISMS

These are the most common hypersensitivity reactions. They are characterized by production of **IgE** antibody directed against harmless environmental antigens, and are responsible for most **allergies**. The antigens involved are called **allergens**, and are often small, **highly soluble proteins** as these characteristics seem to favour a T-helper type 2 (T_H2) response, which is required for IgE production. The route of antigen delivery seems to be significant and many allergens are delivered in small doses through mucosal surfaces, such as the respiratory tract.

Allergic reactions do not occur in all individuals exposed to allergens and some people are more prone to these conditions than others. This characteristic is known as **atopy** and **atopic** individuals produce high levels of IgE to a wide variety of antigens. The reasons for this are not fully understood, but it appears to have a genetic basis.

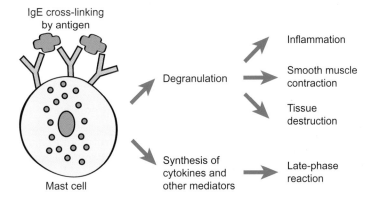

Once produced, IgE molecules bind to the surface of mast cells residing in the tissues. If re-exposure to the allergen occurs, antibody cross-linking induces mast cell **degranulation**, releasing preformed inflammatory mediators, such as **histamine** and **proteases**, into the local environment. These cause inflammation, smooth muscle contraction and tissue destruction. This occurs within minutes of exposure and constitutes the **immediate reaction** in an allergic response.

Furthermore, there is a second stage in an allergic response, known as the **late-phase reaction**, which develops several hours after exposure. This occurs because mast cells are induced to synthesize a variety of cytokines and other inflammatory mediators. These have a number of effects, including recruitment of other cell types, such as eosinophils, basophils and T_H2 cells, which contribute to further tissue damage and IgE production.

Answers
3. T T F T F
4. C, E, B, H, D, F
5. F F T F

6. **Are the following statements relating to anaphylaxis true or false?**

a. It can occur when an allergen is systemically present throughout the bloodstream
b. It is associated with a marked rise in blood pressure
c. It causes swelling of the larynx and results in obstruction to breathing
d. It is most commonly associated with drug allergies
e. It is treated with rapid administration of adrenaline

7. **True or false? Allergic reactions to allergens ingested via the gastrointestinal tract can result in**

a. Diarrhoea
b. Anaphylaxis
c. Vomiting

d. Urticaria
e. Allergic rhinitis

8. **Regarding allergic reactions to inhaled antigens**

a. Allergic rhinitis is caused by degranulation of mast cells associated with the nasal mucosa
b. Allergic rhinitis is associated with decreased mucous production in the nose
c. Pollen is a common allergen causing allergic rhinitis
d. Allergic asthma is associated with relaxation of bronchial smooth muscle
e. Eosinophils are important cells in maintaining inflammation in allergic asthma
f. Allergic asthma is characterized by bronchial hyper-responsiveness to a wide variety of stimuli

9. **Fill in the blanks in the following statements regarding treatment of allergies using the options below (each option can be used once, more than once or not at all)**

Options

A. Corticosteroids
B. Salbutamol

C. Prednisolone
D. Bronchodilators

E. Antihistamines
F. Cetirizine

1. One commonly used group of drugs are _____, which directly block the actions of the inflammatory mediator histamine
2. _____ are commonly used to treat inflammatory allergic conditions, such as asthma
3. _____ are a group of drugs that cause relaxation of bronchial smooth muscle. _____ is an example that is commonly used in asthma

EXPLANATION: TYPE 1 HYPERSENSITIVITY REACTIONS – EXAMPLES AND TREATMENT

Type 1 hypersensitivity reactions can result in a variety of clinical syndromes, depending on the allergen involved and the method of exposure.

The most severe example is known as **anaphylaxis** (or **anaphylactic shock**). This can occur when an allergen is systemically present in the bloodstream. Widespread mast cell degranulation causes vasodilation and increased vascular permeability, resulting in a marked fall in blood pressure and swelling of tissues. Furthermore, airway constriction and swelling of the larynx results in potentially fatal obstruction to breathing. This syndrome must be treated rapidly with injection of **adrenaline** (epinephrine), which causes vasoconstriction and increases cardiac output to maintain blood pressure, and prevents mast cell degranulation. Anaphylaxis is most commonly associated with drug allergies or bee stings, but can also occur in some food allergies.

Most hypersensitivity reactions to allergens ingested via the gastrointestinal tract have less serious consequences. Localized mast cell degranulation causes smooth muscle contraction resulting in **diarrhoea** and **vomiting**. When the allergen is absorbed into the bloodstream, it can activate mast cells in the skin resulting in a widespread **wheal-and-flair** response, known as **urticaria**. This is characterized by erythema associated with raised oedematous lesions.

Another common method of allergen exposure is inhalation, which causes two main syndromes. **Allergic rhinitis** is caused by mast cell degranulation in the nasal mucosa. This causes increased mucous production as well as itching, sneezing and localized oedema. This is commonly a consequence of pollen allergies, when it is known as **hay fever**. The other common syndrome seen is **allergic asthma**, which is characterized by **airway constriction**. Chronic inflammation subsequently ensues, with the continued presence of activated inflammatory cells, particularly eosinophils. The airways become hyper-responsive to a wide variety of stimuli in addition to the initial allergen.

There are a number of treatments used for type 1 hypersensitivity reactions. Common drugs include **antihistamines**, which antagonize the actions of histamine. Anti-inflammatory drugs, such as **corticosteroids**, can be used when inflammation plays an important role, such as in asthma. In addition, **bronchodilators**, such as salbutamol, which cause relaxation of airway smooth muscle, are commonly used in asthma.

Answers

6. T F T T T
7. T T T T F
8. T F T F T T
9. 1 – E; 2 – A; 3 – D, B

10. **Answer the following questions about type 2 hypersensitivity reactions**

    a. List three ways in which antibodies can cause cell damage in type 2 hypersensitivity reactions

    b. Give an example of another way that type 2 hypersensitivity reactions can cause harm, other than by causing damage to cells

    c. Explain the mechanism of drug-induced haemolysis

    d. Give an example of a drug that can cause this condition

11. **Put the following statements regarding haemolytic disease of the newborn in the correct order**

    a. During delivery of her first baby, some fetal erythrocytes pass into the maternal bloodstream during the traumatic events of birth

    b. Anti-rhesus IgG crosses the placenta into the fetal circulation, where it causes haemolysis of the fetal erythrocytes, leading to severe disease and possibly death of the fetus or newborn

    c. The mother's immune system mounts an immune response, resulting in the production of anti-rhesus antibody, including IgG

    d. The mother becomes pregnant for a second time with a rhesus-positive fetus

    e. A rhesus-negative mother becomes pregnant for the first time with a rhesus-positive fetus

12. **How can haemolytic disease of the newborn be prevented?**

ADCC, antibody-dependent cell-mediated cytotoxicity; Ig, immunoglobulin

EXPLANATION: TYPE 2 HYPERSENSITIVITY REACTIONS

These immune responses result in tissue damage due to antibody binding either directly or indirectly to self-cells. Cell damage occurs as a result of antibody effector functions, including **opsonization, antibody-dependent cell-mediated cytotoxicity (ADCC)** and **complement activation**, all of which stimulate inflammation.

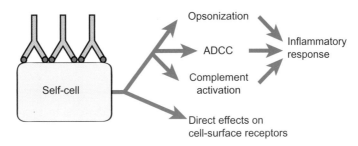

An example of this type of response to an exogenous antigen is **drug-induced haemolysis**. This occurs because certain drugs, such as **penicillin**, bind to the surface of red blood cells **(10c)**. If antibodies are then formed against the drug, they mediate destruction of the cells.

Another example of a type 2 hypersensitivity reaction is **haemolytic disease of the newborn**. This is caused by antibodies targeting the **rhesus D antigen**, which is found on the surface of certain individuals' red blood cells. If a rhesus-negative mother becomes pregnant with a rhesus-positive fetus her immune system can be exposed to the antigen if fetal cells pass into the maternal circulation, such as during the traumatic events of delivery. This stimulates the production of **anti-rhesus antibody** by the mother. If she subsequently has another pregnancy with a rhesus-positive fetus, the IgG antibody produced can cross the placenta and cause haemolysis of the fetal erythrocytes, leading to severe anaemia and, potentially, death. This condition can be prevented by administering anti-rhesus antibody (anti-D) to the mother after delivery of the initial pregnancy **(12)**. This mops up any rhesus antigen that may have passed into the maternal circulation, preventing her immune system being exposed to the antigen and a response being mounted.

Type 2 hypersensitivity reactions are also the mechanism behind many **autoimmune** diseases, in which antibodies are formed against self-antigens, resulting in cell damage. Furthermore, in some autoimmune conditions the antibodies have other harmful effects, such as stimulation of cell-surface receptors, as is the case in Graves' disease.

Answers

10. a – Opsonization, complement activation, Antibody-dependent cell-mediated cytotoxicity; b – Effects on cell-surface receptors; c – See explanation; d – Penicillin

11. e, a, c, d, b

12. See explanation

13. Considering immune complexes

a. Immune complexes are always formed in interactions between antibody and soluble antigens

b. Formation of immune complexes always results in disease

c. Immune complexes are usually removed from the circulation by phagocytes, such as monocytes

d. Some immune complexes can become deposited in the tissues, where they induce an inflammatory response

e. Relative excess of antigen over antibody favours production of immune complexes that can become deposited in the tissues

14. Put the following statements regarding the mechanisms of type 3 hypersensitivity reactions in the correct order

a. Immune complexes bind to Fc receptors on the surfaces of leukocytes and platelets, activating the cells

b. IgG antibody is formed against a soluble antigen

c. Complement activation and release of inflammatory mediators by activated leukocytes and platelets results in an acute inflammatory response

d. Re-exposure to the same antigen results in formation of immune complexes

15. Using the information on the opposite page and the previous page, classify the following conditions as being mediated by which type of hypersensitivity reaction

Options

A. Type 2
B. Type 3

1. Drug-induced haemolysis
2. Arthus reaction
3. Systemic lupus erythematosus
4. Graves' disease
5. Farmer's lung
6. Haemolytic disease of the newborn

Fc, fragment crystallizable; Ig, immunoglobulin

EXPLANATION: TYPE 3 HYPERSENSITIVITY REACTIONS

These occur following formation of **immune complexes** between soluble antigens and antibodies. These complexes are always formed in any interaction between antibody and soluble antigen, but are usually safely removed from the circulation by **phagocytic cells**, such as monocytes. However, under certain circumstances and in certain individuals, they can become deposited in the tissues. This tends to occur when small complexes are formed owing to the relative excess of antigen in comparison to antibody. The complexes can then induce an inflammatory response by activating complement and binding to Fc receptors on leukocytes and platelets, activating the cells.

An example of this is the **Arthus reaction**, in which subcutaneous injection of a soluble antigen into an individual who has previously formed IgG against it results in local inflammation. Another example is the condition **farmer's lung**, in which individuals form IgG against inhaled allergens, such as mould spores. Subsequent re-exposure results in formation of immune complexes in the lungs and eventually permanent tissue damage. Similar mechanisms appear to be responsible for several autoimmune conditions, such as **systemic lupus erythematosus**, in which formation of autoantibodies results in deposition of immune complexes at various sites in the body, including the blood vessels, kidneys and lungs.

Answers
13. T F T T T
14. b, d, a, c
15. 1 – A, 2 – B, 3 – B, 4 – A, 5 – B, 6 – A

16. **Use the options below to fill in the blanks in the following paragraph regarding type 4 hypersensitivity reactions (each option can be used once, more than once or not at all)**

Options

A. Acute
B. Tuberculosis
C. Granuloma
D. Antibody

E. Chronic
F. Cytotoxicity
G. Inflammatory
H. Immediate

I. Delayed
J. T cell
K. Hepatitis B

Type 4 hypersensitivity reactions are conditions in which tissue damage is caused by an inappropriate or excessive _____ response, and are also known as _____-type hypersensitivity reactions. Tissue damage can be caused by release of _____ cytokines and/or cell mediated _____. Examples of these conditions include contact hypersensitivity reactions, as well as some _____ infections, including _____. In the latter example, the immune system is unable to eliminate the pathogen, and persistent T cell responses result in _____ inflammation and _____ formation

17. **Arrange the statements below regarding the mechanisms of a positive tuberculin skin test in the correct order**

   a. Initial exposure to *Mycobacterium tuberculosis* results in an immune response and development of long-lived memory T cells
   b. T_H1 cells proliferate and release inflammatory cytokines
   c. Antigenic peptides from the organism *M. tuberculosis* are injected subcutaneously
   d. Antigenic peptides are taken up by APCs and presented on their surface in conjunction with MHC class II molecules
   e. A visible inflammatory response develops around the injection site around 24 hours after exposure, confirming previous exposure to *M. tuberculosis*
   f. Memory T_H1 cells previously formed against *M. tuberculosis* recognize peptide:MHC class II complexes on the surface of APCs

18. **Concerning contact hypersensitivity reactions**

   a. Contact hypersensitivity reactions can occur to some metals
   b. Contact hypersensitivity reactions can be mediated by either CD4 or CD8 T cells
   c. Pentadecacatechol, found in poison ivy, causes immunogenic modified self-peptides to be presented on the surface of self-cells
   d. Tissue damage in reactions to poison ivy can be caused by cell-mediated cytotoxicity

APC, antigen-presenting cell; MHC, major histocompatibility comlex; T_H1, T-helper type 1

EXPLANATION: TYPE 4 HYPERSENSITIVITY REACTIONS

Type 4 hypersensitivity reactions are characterized by tissue damage as a result of **T cell responses**. The mechanisms of tissue damage can include release of inflammatory cytokines and cell-mediated cytotoxicity. Type 4 hypersensitivity reactions are also known as delayed-type hypersensitivity reactions because the symptoms start to develop about 24 hours after exposure to stimulus.

An example of this type of reaction is the **tuberculin skin test**, which tests for previous exposure to *Mycobacterium tuberculosis*. It involves subcutaneous injection of peptides from the microorganisms. These are taken up and presented by host antigen-presenting cells (APCs) in conjunction with major histocompatibility class (MHC) class II molecules. Individuals who have previously been exposed to *M. tuberculosis* have developed memory T_H1 cells, which recognize these peptide:MHC complexes and release inflammatory cytokines. This results in a visible inflammatory response after 24 hours, which confirms previous exposure to *M. tuberculosis*.

Similar mechanisms are responsible for many **contact hypersensitivity** reactions, which can be caused by a variety of substances, including some metals such as nickel. These can be either CD4 or CD8 cell-mediated. An example of a CD8 cell-mediated reaction is the response to poison ivy. This plant contains **pentadecacatechol**, which passes into host cells, where it modifies host proteins, resulting in the presentation of antigenic peptides within MHC class I molecules. These are then recognized by CD8 T cells, which kill the cell and release inflammatory cytokines.

Type 4 hypersensitivity reactions are also responsible for tissue damage in a number of chronic infections, such as tuberculosis. In this situation, the immune system is unable to eliminate the pathogen, and the continued T cell response results in chronic inflammation, leading to tissue destruction and granuloma formation.

Answers
16. J, I, G, F, E, B, E, C
17. a, c, d, f, b, e
18. T T T T

19. Regarding autoimmunity

a. Controlled self-reactive immune cells can be found in a normal immune system
b. Self-reactive immune cells never cause disease
c. Autoimmune disease is multifactorial in origin
d. The surrounding environment does not have a role in autoimmune disease development
e. Genetic make-up has a role in autoimmune disease development

20. How have monozygotic twin studies shown the importance of genetic make-up in autoimmune disease?

21. Which major histocompatibility complex alleles are associated with the following autoimmune diseases?

a. Rheumatoid arthritis
b. Ankylosing spondylitis

22. Fill in the blanks in the following paragraph concerning autoimmunity using the options below (each option can be used once, more than once or not at all)

Options

A. Autoantibody
B. Central nervous system
C. Lungs
D. Autoantigen

E. Myelin sheaths
F. Limb weakness
G. Visual disturbance

An autoimmune response is triggered by immune recognition of an _____, the location of which often determines resulting disease. This is demonstrated in a disease involving the _____ called multiple sclerosis. Multiple sclerosis sufferers report symptoms including _____ and _____. These symptoms result from autoimmune destruction of the _____ surrounding nerves in the brain and spinal cord

23. Describe the phenomenon of determinant spreading

HLA, human leukocyte antigen; MHC, major histocompatibility complex

EXPLANATION: AUTOIMMUNITY

Autoimmunity refers to the attack of self-tissues by the immune system. Naturally self-reactive T and B cells are found in a normal healthy immune system, where they perform functions including the scavenging of senescent cells. However, it is widely accepted that uncontrolled autoreactive immune components can also damage tissues and organs leading to **autoimmune disease**. Autoimmune disease is characterized by the presence of activated **self-reactive T cells** and **autoantibodies**. It is believed to be multifactorial in origin, with contributory factors including genetic predisposition and the surrounding environment.

The importance of **genetic predisposition** has been shown by a high rate of **concordance** in monozygotic twins **(20)**. Accordingly, it has been observed that some **human leukocyte antigen (HLA) alleles** occur at higher frequencies in people with specific autoimmune diseases compared to the general population. For example, the MHC class II allele **HLA-DR4** is associated with **rheumatoid arthritis** development, and the MHC class I allele **HLA-B27** is associated with an 80-fold increased risk of developing **ankylosing spondylitis**. Specific HLA association with autoimmunity may reflect differences in negative selection in the thymus and peptide presentation in the periphery. For example, it is possible that HLA-B27 alleles present the spinal cartilage antigens targeted in ankylosing spondylitis very efficiently to T cells. In addition, environmental signals, such as the presence of concurrent infection, will influence the development of autoimmunity by altering both reactivity of the immune system and the susceptibility of different tissues to attack.

The initial trigger for an autoimmune response is recognition of a self-antigen (also known as an **autoantigen**). The location of these autoantigens often determines resulting disease. This is demonstrated in a disease involving the central nervous system called **multiple sclerosis**. Multiple sclerosis is commonly characterized by development of scattered symptoms, including limb weakness, numbness and tingling, and visual disturbances. These symptoms directly result from autoimmune destruction of the myelin sheaths surrounding different nerves in the brain and spinal cord.

As self-cells are damaged and their contents released, antigens that are usually hidden become visible to the immune system. These new autoantigens stimulate more peripheral autoreactive T cells, leading to further tissue damage. This phenomenon contributes to autoimmune disease propagation and is called **determinant spreading (23)**.

Answers

19. T F T F T
20. See explanation
21. a – HLA-DR4, b – HLA-B27
22. D, B, F, G, E
23. See explanation

24. Name two main tolerance components that autoreactive cells must survive in order to initiate autoimmunity

 25. Answer the following questions using statements from the list below (each option can be used once, more than once or not at all)

Options

A. Molecular mimicry
B. Weak avidity interaction
C. Bystander activation
D. Mutation in genes responsible for T cell apoptosis
E. Isoform absence in the thymus
F. Autoantigen absence in the thymus

1. These theories propose pathogen presence can initiate autoimmune disease
2. These theories explain escape of central tolerance by self-reactive T cells
3. This can explain the observed association between certain MHC alleles and autoimmune disease.
4. This may explain the association between Coxsackie B4 virus and type 1 diabetes mellitus
5. This is minimized by promiscuous gene expression in thymic epithelial cells
6. This involves cross-reaction between microbial and host antigens
7. This involves alteration in the processing and presentation of self-antigen by APCs

APC, antigen-presenting cell; MHC, major histocompatibility complex; TCR, T cell receptor

EXPLANATION: MECHANISMS OF AUTOIMMUNITY

Autoimmunity involves the **breakdown** of **immune tolerance**. Thus, modulation or interference with tolerance mechanisms will allow autoreactive T cells to escape from the thymus and survive in the periphery. Although autoreactive B cells often contribute to autoimmune disease, the importance of T cells in promoting B cell responses means that loss of T cell tolerance is more significant.

Avoiding central tolerance: Various mechanisms allow self-reactive cells to escape central tolerance mediated by the thymus. For example, **absence** of an **autoantigen** in the thymus will result in **avoidance** of **negative selection**. As mentioned before, this is limited by promiscuous thymic gene expression, which means developing T cells are exposed to a large range of self-antigens. It is also possible that the autoantigen responsible for an autoimmune lesion may be present in the thymus but may be found in the periphery as a **different isoform** able to activate T cells. Additionally, if **interaction** of the specific TCR with self-antigen:MHC is too **weak**, negative selection may fail. In other words, weak unstable binding may mean autoreactive T cells are not deleted. This is one possible explanation for the observed association between autoimmune disease and certain MHC alleles. Negative selection of the T cell repertoire can also be altered by genetic **mutation**. For example, mutations in genes encoding molecules involved in apoptosis may mean self-reactive T cells are not eliminated.

Avoiding peripheral tolerance: Peripheral tolerance mechanisms are important when central tolerance mechanisms fail to purge the T cell repertoire of autoreactivity. However, they too can be avoided. It has been suggested that microbial agents or viruses can contain structures that mimic normal host self-proteins in structure or sequence. Following infection, T and B cells specific for these microbial antigens are activated. Consequently, the activated cells can cross-react with host proteins and cause autoimmune destruction. This theory is termed **molecular mimicry**. Infection can also change the peripheral **cytokine environment**. It has been proposed that APCs may alter the processing and presentation of self-antigen to potentially self-reactive T cells in the presence of inflammatory mediators induced by a pathogen. This concept is known as **bystander activation**. It is thought to play a role in the observed association between Coxsackie B4 virus and type 1 diabetes mellitus.

Answers

24. Central tolerance and peripheral tolerance
25. 1 – A, C; 2 – B, D, E, F; 3 – B; 4 – C; 5 – F; 6 – A; 7 – C

26. True or false? The following autoimmune diseases are primarily mediated by antibodies

    a. Myasthenia gravis
    b. Systemic lupus erythematosus
    c. Multiple sclerosis
    d. Graves' disease
    e. Insulin-dependent diabetes mellitus

27. Name autoimmune diseases that target the following self-antigens

    a. Myelin proteins
    b. Pancreatic β cells
    c. Systemic DNA

28. A 60-year-old woman arrives in clinic. She describes a 2-month history of swollen, painful fingers in both hands. You take a blood sample. Your findings help to confirm a diagnosis of rheumatoid arthritis

    a. What autoantibody did you find in her blood?
    b. Her mother had 'joint problems' and family studies of rheumatoid arthritis have shown high concordance rates in monozygotic twins. What does this mean?
    c. Although T and B cells are implicated in initiating rheumatoid arthritis, what two factors are responsible for her joint damage?

DNA, deoxyribonucleic acid; Ig, immunoglobulin; TSH, thyroid stimulating hormone

EXPLANATION: AUTOIMMUNE DISEASE

Autoimmune diseases and consequent tissue damage may be predominantly **antibody** or **cell mediated** (see table below for some examples).

Main mediator of damage	Disease	Target	Result
Antibody	Graves' disease	Thyroid-stimulating hormone receptor	Thyroid overactivity leading to goitre, opthalmopathy and systemic symptoms
	Myasthenia gravis	Nicotinic acetylcholine receptor	Muscle weakness
	Systemic lupus erythematosus	DNA, histones, ribosomes	Immune complex deposition leads to glomerulonephritis, vasculitis, arthritis
T cells	Multiple sclerosis	Myelin proteins	Limb numbness, weakness, tingling
	Insulin-dependent diabetes mellitus	Pancreatic β cells	Insulin deficiency

Although the specific autoimmune disease mechanism may be mainly antibody- or cell-mediated, it is important to remember that B cells do not produce significant antibody levels unless they receive some initial T cell help. Often, T and B cells may be specifically implicated in autoimmune damage together. For example, in **Hashimoto's thyroiditis**, both antibody and T cells attack antigens within the thyroid gland, leading to thyroid destruction and often hypothyroidism. By contrast, in **Graves' disease**, an IgG antibody directed against the TSH-receptor expressed by thyroid follicular cells stimulates thyroid hormone production leading to hyperthyroidism.

Another relatively common disorder thought to have an autoimmune pathogenesis is **rheumatoid arthritis**, a disease of the synovial lining of joints. Sufferers commonly report swollen, painful and stiff fingers, wrists and ankles. Symptoms can fluctuate, and further joints, such as the cervical spine, are often involved. The immune responses and specific self-antigens involved in rheumatoid arthritis have not been conclusively demonstrated. However, **infiltrates of activated T cells** are usually seen within the inflamed joint synovium. Additionally, about 80 per cent of cases are seropositive for **rheumatoid factor** produced by B cells. Rheumatoid factor represents an autoantibody directed at antigenic epitopes present on existing IgG. Although both T and B cells appear to have a role in initiating autoimmunity, the actual damage to joints and extra-articular structures is due to resultant formation of an **inflammatory granulation tissue** called **pannus**. This spreads over and gradually erodes the cartilage and bone of the joint. Additionally, granulomatous lesions, called **rheumatoid nodules,** are found in extra-articular sites, such as the pleura and pericardium.

As autoimmune disease is caused by the action of normal immune mechanisms, controlling and treating disease without vastly increasing susceptibility of the patient to infection is important. Classes of **immuno-suppressive drugs** that are used include **anti-inflammatory** agents, such as corticosteroids, **cytotoxic** agents, such as azathioprine, and drugs that **inhibit T cell activation**, such as cyclosporin A.

Answers

26. T T F T F
27. a – Multiple sclerosis, b – Diabetes mellitus, c – Systemic lupus erythematosus
28. a – High levels of rheumatoid factor, b – There is an important inherited genetic susceptibility to rheumatoid arthritis, c – Inflammation and pannus formation

29. Concerning immunodeficiency disorders

    a. Immunodeficiencies can predispose to certain tumours
    b. Disorders affecting T cells tend to predispose to infection with pyogenic bacteria
    c. Disorders affecting B cells predispose primarily to viral infection
    d. Primary immunodeficiencies have a genetic basis
    e. Secondary immunodeficiencies can be caused by infection

30. With regard to severe combined immunodeficiency

    a. This is a consequence of disordered development of both B and T cells
    b. It is always inherited by an X-linked pattern
    c. Presentation usually occurs in late childhood
    d. It can cause failure to thrive in infants
    e. Treatment with immunoglobulin replacement therapy can be successful

31. A 10-month-old boy has been suffering from recurrent respiratory tract and skin infections for the last six months. During one episode, *Streptococcus pneumoniae* is cultured from a sputum sample. His serum immunoglobulin (Ig)G level is found to be markedly reduced, while IgM and IgA levels are undetectable

    a. Name a primary immunodeficiency that could account for these findings
    b. What type of cell is affected in this condition and what is the cause?
    c. How can it be treated?
    d. Give two examples of other conditions affecting antibody production

32. Considering primary immunodeficiencies affecting T cells

    a. These are the most common primary immunodeficiencies
    b. They typically predispose to intracellular infections
    c. Failure of development of the thymus is characteristic of DiGeorge syndrome
    d. DiGeorge syndrome characteristically results in markedly decreased immunoglobulin levels
    e. DiGeorge syndrome is associated with impaired development of the parathyroid glands

33. Give an example of a primary immunodeficiency disease caused by a defect in the innate immune system

CVID, common variable immunodeficiency; Ig, immunoglobulin; SCID, severe combined immunodeficiency

EXPLANATION: IMMUNODEFICIENCIES

Defects in the immune system can result in increased susceptibility to infection and certain tumours, and are known as **immunodeficiency diseases**. The consequences of these disorders depend on the components of the immune system affected. Defects in antibody production predispose to infections by pyogenic bacteria, as opsonization by antibody is critical in clearing these infections. Defects of T cell function primarily predispose to infection with intracellular pathogens. Immunodeficiencies can be classified as **primary**, which have a genetic basis, or **secondary**, which are caused by processes such as infection or nutritional deficiencies.

Primary immunodeficiencies: The most severe disorders affect development of both B and T cells, and result in a condition called **severe combined immunodeficiency (SCID)**. There are a number of genetic defects that cause this condition, which can be inherited in X-linked or autosomal patterns. SCID presents in the first few months of life with persistent infections and **failure to thrive**, and is fatal within a few years unless treated with bone marrow transplantation.

There are several conditions that affect B cell function. **X-linked agammaglobulinaemia**, for instance, is caused by a deficiency in B cell tyrosine kinase, which has a role in B cell development **(31b)**. It results in very low counts of immunoglobulins in the blood and presents with recurrent bacterial infections after about four months of life. It can be treated with immunoglobulin replacement therapy **(31c)**. Other disorders of antibody production include **common variable immunodeficiency (CVID)**, a heterogeneous group of antibody deficiencies, and selective **IgA deficiency (31d)**.

Primary immunodeficiencies primarily affecting T cell function are rare. The commonest example is **DiGeorge syndrome**, which is caused by **impaired development** of the **thymus**, **parathyroid glands** and **great vessels**. It results in markedly decreased T cell numbers, leading to increased susceptibility to intracellular infections, while antibody levels are often normal.

Several immunodeficiencies are caused by defects in the innate immune system. Examples include various **complement deficiencies** and **chronic granulomatous disease**, which is caused by impaired phagocyte function **(31)**.

Answers
29. T F F T T
30. T F F T F
31. a – X-linked agammaglobulinaemia; b, c, d – See explanation
32. F T T F T
33. See explanation

34. Case history: A 25-year-old man experienced a brief flu-like illness shortly after having unprotected sex. This illness resolved and he remained well for 7 years subsequently, after which he began to experience recurrent oral candidiasis. A few months later, he developed a productive cough, fever and malaise. Acid-fast bacilli were detected in his sputum and a diagnosis of pulmonary tuberculosis was made

    a. What virus is likely to be the underlying cause of these symptoms?
    b. What cell types are infected by this virus and how does it infect them?
    c. What is the asymptomatic phase of this condition known as and what happens during this period to the CD4 T cell count in the blood?

    It is suspected that the above patient may be suffering from a form of immunodeficiency and, after appropriate counselling, he agrees to undergo an HIV test. Anti-HIV IgM and IgG are detected in his serum, confirming HIV infection. At this time, his CD4 T cell count is found to be 189/μL.

    d. What is the name of the immunodeficiency from which this man is suffering?
    e. What other types of infections is he likely to be susceptible to as his condition progresses?
    f. Other than these infections, what other conditions are often seen in AIDS patients?
    g. What treatment is available to slow the progression of AIDS, and what is its major drawback?
    h. What methods could potentially reduce the spread of HIV worldwide, both now and in the future?

35. Answer the following questions regarding HIV infection using the options below

Options

A. Pox virus	**F.** 1200/μL	**K.** *Pneumocystis carinii* pneumonia
B. Tuberculosis	**G.** Cytomegalovirus	**L.** Adenovirus
C. CD8	**H.** gp120	**M.** Oral candidiasis
D. Retrovirus	**I.** 200/μL	**N.** CD4
E. Provirus	**J.** Rhinovirus	

1. What type of virus is HIV?
2. Which glycoprotein on host cells does HIV bind to?
3. What is the virus known as during the time when its genome is integrated into the host cell DNA?
4. At what CD4 count does the infected individual become susceptible to opportunistic pathogens?
5. Name two infections commonly seen early in the course of AIDS

AIDS, acquired immunodeficiency syndrome; DNA, deoxyribonucleic acid; HIV, human immunodeficiency virus; Ig, immunoglobulin; RNA, ribonucleic acid

EXPLANATION: SECONDARY IMMUNODEFICIENCY – HIV AND AIDS

The most important secondary immunodeficiency disorder is the **acquired immunodeficiency syndrome** (AIDS) **(34d)**, caused by the **human immunodeficiency virus** (HIV) **(34a)**. HIV is a **retrovirus**, composed of two copies of its RNA genome within a protein core, surrounded by a lipid membrane envelope containing the glycoproteins gp120 and gp41. The virus infects cells expressing **surface CD4**, importantly including CD4 T cells. The glycoprotein gp120 binds CD4, and gp41 facilitates fusion of the envelope with the cell membrane, allowing entry of the virus **(34b)**. DNA is then formed from viral RNA by the enzyme **reverse transcriptase**. This DNA integrates into the host cell DNA, where it is known as a **provirus**. Subsequent transcription of viral DNA results in formation of new virus particles.

HIV infection occurs by exposure to infected body fluids, commonly by sexual intercourse or use of contaminated needles, and also by vertical transmission from mother to child. After an initial flu-like illness an immune response controls but cannot eliminate the infection. There follows an asymptomatic period of about 2–12 years, known as **clinical latency**, during which viral replication continues and the CD4 T cell count in the blood falls **(34c)**. When the CD4 cell count reaches about 200/µL (normal levels are about 1200/µL) the individual becomes susceptible to **opportunistic infections** and can be considered to have developed AIDS, which causes death within 20 months, if untreated.

The initial infections seen include **oral candidiasis** and **tuberculosis**. As the disease progresses and the CD4 cell count falls, individuals become susceptible to less virulent organisms, such as **cytomegalovirus**, **atypical mycobacteria** and the fungus *Pneumocystis carinii*, which causes severe pneumonia **(34e)**. Certain malignancies caused by oncogenic viruses are common, including **B cell lymphomas** and **Kaposi's sarcoma**. Patients also often suffer a wasting syndrome and a minority develop dementia caused by infection of microglial cells in the brain **(34f)**.

Drugs that **inhibit retroviral enzymes** are available and can slow progression of the disease. However, these are very expensive, so are not practical in the developing world **(34g)**. Research into vaccine development is under way, with novel techniques showing potential. However, the most effective methods currently available to limit spread of the disease are **public health measures**, including education on safer sex **(34h)**.

Answers
34. See explanation
35. 1 – D; 2 – N; 3 – E; 4 – I; 5 – B, M

36. Regarding acquired immunodeficiency

a. Malnutrition is the most common cause of secondary immunodeficiency
b. Protein deficiency is the most important factor in immune depression owing to malnutrition
c. Nutritional deficiency may enhance cytokine production and antibody secretion
d. Nutritional deficiency may reduce phagocyte function
e. Immunodeficiency due to malnutrition is irreversible
f. Ageing causes an increase in immune responses to exogenous antigens
g. Ageing may cause an increase in autoimmune reactivity
h. Ageing is usually accompanied by reduction in lymphocyte number
i. Immunodeficiency may be seen following measles infection

37. Fill in the blanks in the following paragraph concerning secondary immunodeficiencies using the options below (each option can be used once, more than once or not at all)

Options

A. Leukaemia
B. Rheumatoid arthritis
C. Bone marrow
D. Haematological

E. Malnutrition
F. Lymphoma
G. Infection
H. Myeloma

_____ disorders can suppress production of normal blood cells. _____ involves the unrestricted proliferation of immature leukocytes. This leads to _____ dysfunction and increased susceptibility to _____. Other malignancies involving the bone marrow and secondary lymphoid tissues, such as _____ and _____, will also lead to secondary immunodeficiency

38. Answer the following questions about acquired immunodeficiency owing to the use of certain therapeutic drugs

a. When might immunosuppressive drugs be used?
b. How do some chemotherapy drugs cause increased susceptibility to infection?

39. You are asked to see an 85-year-old patient who is receiving chemotherapy as treatment for leukaemia. Before seeing her, you think about her susceptibility to opportunistic infection. What factors may be important?

AIDS, acquired immunodeficiency syndrome; APC, antigen-presenting cell; HIV, human immunodeficiency virus

EXPLANATION: SECONDARY IMMUNODEFICIENCIES

Acquired, or secondary, immunodeficiencies are considerably more common than primary immuno-deficiencies. Although the best-known cause of secondary immunodeficiency is HIV/AIDS, other causes are important in many patients.

Malnutrition is the leading cause of secondary, or acquired, immunodeficiency. It is well established that nutritional deficiency, particularly **protein shortage**, is strongly associated with impaired immune responses, including reduced phagocyte function, cytokine production and antibody secretion. This is mostly **reversible** upon improvement of nutritional status.

Ageing: Advancing age is associated with immune depression. Paradoxically, it has been observed that ageing involves a **decline in immune responses to exogenous antigens**, but a concurrent **increase in autoimmune reactivity**. The latter occurs despite reductions in lymphocyte number and activity seen with increasing age. Components of the innate immune response also deteriorate with age, e.g. the cough reflex may become less effective at protecting the lower airways from inhaled pathogens.

Infection: Illness, particularly if prolonged and severe, can lead to immune system impairment in a previously healthy individual. Specific infections that cause some immunodeficiency include **infectious mononucleosis, measles** and **chickenpox**. Immunodeficiency following measles infection, for example, is transient and related to viral action on APCs.

Haematological disorders can suppress the production of normal blood cells. For example, **leukaemia** involves the unrestricted proliferation of non-functional immature leukocytes, which compete with normal cells and lead to bone marrow dysfunction. This reduces production of normal leukocytes and causes considerably increased susceptibility to infection. Other malignancies involving the bone marrow and secondary lymphoid tissues, such as **myeloma** and **lymphoma**, will also lead to acquired immunodeficiency.

Drugs: Acquired iatrogenic immunodeficiency may result from use of certain therapeutic drugs. For example, **immunosuppressant** drugs, such as prednisolone, are frequently used following organ transplantation and in treatment of various inflammatory and autoimmune diseases **(38a)**. Such therapy is associated with an increased incidence of opportunistic infection. In addition, many **chemotherapy** drugs used in the treatment of cancer are potent myelosuppressants, which means they reduce blood cell production by the bone marrow **(38b)**. Again, this leads to heightened susceptibility to infection.

Answers

36. T T F T F F T T T
37. D, A, C, G, H, F
38. See explanation
39. Her age, leukaemia and leukaemia chemotherapy may all contribute to reduced immune function

40. Match the following definitions of transplantation types

Options

A. Xenogeneic   C. Autologous
B. Allogeneic   D. Syngeneic

1. Between different sites on the same individual
2. Between genetically unrelated individuals of the same species
3. Between genetically identical individuals
4. Between different species

41. Regarding transplantation

a. Transplant rejection is primarily due to neutrophil action
b. Transplant rejection is primarily due to T cell activation
c. Matching HLA alleles between donor and recipient increases the chance of transplant rejection
d. Differences in minor histocompatibility antigens can cause transplant rejection
e. Minor histocompatibility antigens are identical between members of one species
f. Allogeneic transplantation needs to be followed by immunosuppressive treatment

42. Match the following definitions of transplant rejection types

Options

A. Hyperacute   B. Acute   C. Chronic

1. This is due to targeting by host CD4 and CD8 T cells
2. This is due to pre-existing host antibodies
3. This is due to inflammatory obliteration of vasculature

43. A 25-year-old girl arrives in your clinic. Four weeks ago, she received an allogeneic bone marrow transplant as treatment for leukaemia. She explains that she has had diarrhoea and a painful rash on the palms of her hands for the past couple of weeks

a. What may explain her new symptoms?
b. Why has this occurred?
c. What would be your next step?

GVHD, graft-versus-host disease; HLA, human leukocyte antigen; MHC, major histocompatibility complex

EXPLANATION: TRANSPLANTATION

Transplantation of almost any vital organ or tissue is now well recognized as an effective therapy in many medical conditions. Transplants can be classed as **autologous** (between different sites on the same individual), **syngeneic** (between genetically identical individuals), **allogeneic** (between genetically different individuals of the same species) or, rarely, **xenogeneic** (between different species).

An **acquired immune response** to transplanted tissue is usually the major barrier to successful transplantation. Transplant **rejection** results from **recognition of foreign MHC** by host T cells and subsequent immune activation. Thus, autologous or syngeneic grafts will never be rejected. However, allogeneic grafts, known as allografts, can potentially carry a high risk of rejection. In this case, transplant survival is improved by using a donor with HLA alleles that are as closely matched as possible to recipient alleles. However, lack of donors and extensive HLA polymorphism mean MHC matching may not be complete. Additionally, genetic differences at other loci, such as **minor histocompatibility antigen** loci, can still trigger rejection, albeit more slowly than that seen in MHC-disparate transplants. Minor histocompatibility antigens are polymorphic proteins that differ between members of a species. They are processed by cells and presented by MHC class I molecules. In most cases, **immunosuppressive drugs,** such as **azathioprine** and **cyclosporin A,** help to prevent transplantation rejection.

Rejection of a transplant can be classified as hyperacute, acute or chronic. **Hyperacute rejection** occurs very rapidly and is due to damage by pre-existing host antibodies attacking the transplanted organ. **Acute rejection** is seen within days or weeks, and involves the targeting of transplanted tissue by both CD4 and CD8 host T cells. **Chronic rejection** occurs months to years post-transplant and is due to the progressive inflammatory obliteration of graft vasculature.

The opposite of transplantation rejection is seen in **graft-versus-host disease (GVHD).** This may occur several weeks after allogeneic bone marrow transplantation despite immunosuppressive treatment. Here, the bone marrow graft is immunologically competent and contains T cells able to recognize the recipient's tissues as foreign and mediate an immune reaction to the host **(43b).** Hallmarks of GVHD include a painful **erythematous rash, intestinal injury** and **liver disease.** Treatment involves increasing immunosuppressive therapy.

Answers
40. 1 – C, 2 – B, 3 – D, 4 – A
41. F T F T F T
42. 1 – B, 2 – A, 3 – C
43. a – Graft-versus-host disease, b – See explanation, c – Increase immunosuppressive therapy

44. Fill in the blanks in the following statements concerning vaccination using the options below (each option can be used once, more than once or not at all)

Options

A. Cowpox   **F.** Memory cells
B. Protective immunity   **G.** B cells
C. Smallpox   **H.** Vaccination
D. Hypersensitivity   **I.** *Vaccinia*
E. *Varicella*   **J.** Chickenpox

1. The ability of the immune system to prevent or reduce the level of disease when exposure to a pathogen occurs is known as _____
2. Protection from infection by pathogens to which the immune system has already been exposed is achieved by the development of _____
3. The process used to induce protective immunity to a pathogen without the need for initial infection is known as _____
4. The first successful vaccine was developed by Edward Jenner in 1796 against _____
5. This first vaccine involved inoculation with the _____ virus, which causes the bovine disease _____

45. Concerning the protection conferred by a good vaccine

a. The type of immune response generated often determines the efficacy of a vaccine
b. The ideal vaccine for most intracellular pathogens induces primarily antibody responses
c. The ideal vaccine for most extracellular pathogens induces primarily CD8 T cell responses
d. The ideal vaccine is long lasting, providing lifelong protective immunity to a pathogen without the need for booster vaccines
e. The best possible protection is often achieved if the vaccine is administered by the same route used by the pathogen for infection

46. Discuss the importance of the following factors in the development of a vaccine

a. Safety
b. Practical considerations

Ig, immunoglobulin

EXPLANATION: VACCINATION

When infection with a pathogen occurs, the immune system mounts a response to eliminate the pathogen, followed by development of long-lived **memory cells**. These memory cells can result in **protective immunity**, as a rapid and effective immune response prevents or reduces the severity of disease should re-exposure occur. The aim of **vaccination** is to induce protective immunity without the need for initial infection.

This concept was first developed by **Edward Jenner** in 1796, when he discovered that protective immunity against smallpox could be induced by immunizing individuals with material from pustules from the bovine disease, cowpox, caused by the *Vaccinia* virus. This occurs because this virus contains antigens also present in the smallpox virus. Consequently, memory cells are formed that also protect against smallpox. Subsequently, improved understanding of the immune system has allowed the development of many further vaccines.

A good vaccine should have a number of characteristics, as follows:

- **Protection:** Vaccines should confer good protection against a disease. This involves inducing an appropriate immune response for the pathogen. For example, a good vaccine against an intracellular pathogen should induce development of **memory T cells**, allowing a cell-mediated response, whereas an antibody response is better for most extracellular pathogens. Furthermore, the protection should be **long lasting**, so that booster vaccinations are not required.

    A good vaccine also induces protective responses at appropriate anatomical sites. This is best achieved by administering the vaccine by a **similar route** to that used by the pathogen for infection. For example, the live (Sabin) polio vaccine is administered orally and confers good protection from the disease, which is spread by the faecal–oral route. This is because it induces IgA production along the mucosal surfaces of the gut.
- **Safety (46a):** It is of critical importance that a vaccine does not itself cause disease and that **side-effects** are kept to a minimum.
- **Practical considerations (46b):** A good vaccine should be **inexpensive, easily administered** and **stable** on storage and transport. This allows administration to the maximum number of individuals, including those in rural areas with minimal specialist medical expertise.

Answers
44. 1 – B; 2 – F; 3 – H; 4 – C; 5 – I, A
45. T F F T T
46. See explanation

47. Fill in the blanks in the following statements regarding live, attenuated vaccines using the options below (each option can be used once, more than once or not at all)

Options

A. Virulence   **F.** Genetic engineering

B. Attenuation   **G.** Mutations

C. Able   **H.** Unable

D. Hepatitis   **I.** Tetanus

E. Measles

1. The process of altering an organism to reduce its ability to cause disease is known as _____

2. Attenuation is usually achieved by prolonged culturing of organisms *in vitro*, allowing _____ to develop

3. Future methods of attenuation may include _____, involving direct alteration of a pathogen's DNA

4. An example of a disease for which there is an effective live attenuated vaccine is _____

5. An important characteristic of live attenuated vaccines is that they are _____ to replicate within the host

48. Discuss the advantages and disadvantages of using live attenuated organisms as vaccines

49. Killed organism vaccines

a. Are less likely to cause disease than those using attenuated organisms

b. Provide a sustained source of antigen to the immune system for some time after vaccination

c. Offer an effective means of developing cell mediated memory responses

d. Are of most benefit when an antibody response provides sufficient protection from a pathogen

e. Are used in the Sabin polio vaccine

DNA, deoxyribonucleic acid; MHC, major histocompatibility complex

EXPLANATION: VACCINE STRATEGIES I

There are several strategies that can be used for development of vaccines outlined below.

Live attenuated organisms: One very effective method is the administration of live organisms that have been altered to reduce their virulence. The process of making the organism safe (less virulent) is known as **attenuation** and is usually achieved by prolonged culturing of the organism *in vitro*, allowing mutations to develop. This method has been used to develop vaccines for tuberculosis, polio (the Sabin vaccine), measles, mumps and rubella. In the future, it may be possible to attenuate organisms by directly altering their DNA through genetic engineering.

The advantage of live vaccines is that they have similar characteristics to the pathogen so they induce the appropriate type of immune response **(48)**. They are able to replicate and provide a **sustained source of antigen** for the immune system, allowing time for the responses to develop. This can occur at the **same anatomical site** as infection, allowing responses to develop in the appropriate areas. Furthermore, intracellular organisms can replicate within cells, allowing antigens to be presented by MHC class I molecules. This allows the development of CD8 memory T cells.

The main drawback of live attenuated vaccines is the risk that they may **cause disease (48)**. This can occur if the organisms undergo further mutations and regain their virulence. Furthermore, even without further mutations, attenuated vaccines can potentially cause disease in immunocompromised individuals.

Killed organisms: Another strategy is the administration of whole microorganisms that have been treated to stop them being able to replicate. These are generally safer than attenuated vaccines, as they are unable to cause disease, although there have been concerns that some do have side-effects. Disadvantages include the fact that they cannot provide a sustained source of antigen and that as no antigen is produced within host cells, they are unable to induce CD8 T cell responses. They can, however, be effective when an antibody response alone is adequate. This type of vaccine has been developed against rabies, polio (the Salk vaccine) and pertussis (whooping cough).

Answers

47. 1 – B, 2 – G, 3 – F, 4 – E, 5 – C
48. See explanation
49. T F F T F

50. Subunit vaccines

a. Can occasionally cause disease
b. Tend to be of high immunogenicity
c. Often need to be given with adjuvants
d. For hepatitis B are effective in all individuals
e. Have the disadvantage of relying on immune responses to a single antigen

51. Fill in the blanks in the following statements using the options provided (each option can be used once, more than once or not at all)

Options

A. Alum
B. Lipopolysaccharide
C. IgG
D. DNA
E. Toxin
F. T-helper
G. IgM

H. Pathogens
I. DNA vaccines
J. Conjugate
K. Harmless
L. Adjuvants
M. Toxoid
N. Capsular polysaccharide

1. The *Haemophilus influenzae* type B vaccine is a type of subunit vaccine known as a _____ vaccine. It is composed of _____ bound to bacterial proteins. It induces production of _____ as the bacterial proteins initiate a _____ cell response, which allows appropriate antibody production by B cells
2. The main cause of pathology in tetanus is _____ production. The vaccine for this disease is a type of subunit vaccine, known as a _____ vaccine. This is an inactivated form of the _____, which induces long-standing _____ production. Any _____ produced on subsequent exposure to the pathogen is, therefore, quickly neutralized
3. Substances added to vaccines to increase their immunogenicity are known as _____. The only example currently in use in humans is _____
4. Prospects for future vaccine development include the use of _____ microbes, which have been modified to express antigens from _____
5. Another potential future development is the use of _____, which involve administration of _____ encoding pathogenic antigens. This becomes transcribed by host cells, resulting in an immune response to the antigen

---

APC, antigen presenting cell; DNA, deoxyribonucleic acid; Ig, immunoglobulin

EXPLANATION: VACCINE STRATEGIES II

Subunit vaccines: Another strategy is to administer subunits of microorganisms containing **immunogenic antigens**. These are safe, as the vaccine cannot cause disease. However, they tend to be of low immunogenicity and often have to be given with adjuvants (see below) to increase the immune response.

An example of this type of vaccine is the hepatitis B vaccine, which consists of the surface antigen of the virus and induces IgG production. However, it is ineffective in certain individuals, possibly because their APCs are unable to present the antigen. This is one disadvantage of subunit vaccines, as they rely on responses to a **single antigen** rather than a whole organism containing several antigens.

Subunit vaccines have been developed against a number of bacteria, including *Streptococcus pneumoniae* and *Haemophilus influenzae* type B. They induce antibody production against bacterial capsular polysaccharides, allowing opsonization of the bacteria. However, polysaccharides alone cannot induce IgG production, as they do not initiate T-helper cell responses. They are, therefore, often given conjugated to bacterial proteins, allowing T-helper cells to be activated. Consequently, they are known as **conjugate vaccines**.

Another type of subunit vaccine can give protection against bacterial diseases for which the main cause of pathology is toxin production, such as tetanus and diphtheria. By administering an inactivated form of the toxin, known as a **toxoid**, an IgG response can be induced. Consequently, on subsequent exposure to the pathogen, any toxin produced is neutralized.

Adjuvants: These are substances that are added to vaccines to increase their immunogenicity. They can work in a number of ways, including induction of **inflammation** and **cytokine** production, and by concentrating the antigen in appropriate sites. The only adjuvant currently licensed for use in humans is alum, a mixture of aluminium salts.

Future developments: Possible future strategies include the use of harmless microbes genetically modified to produce antigens from pathogenic organisms. Another prospect is vaccination with DNA encoding pathogenic antigens. These **DNA vaccines** can be transcribed and then translated by host cells, inducing an immune response to the encoded protein antigen.

Answers
50. F F T F T
51. 1 – J, N, C, F; 2 – E, M, E, C, E; 3 – L, A; 4 – K, H; 5 – I, D

INDEX